KNOWLEDGE OF HEALTH

The Miseducation of Dieting

T. M. 'Lijah

ISBN-13: 9798650201151

Cover design by: bazz_graphics
Library of Congress Control Number: 2018675309
Printed in the United States of America

This book is dedicated to my mother,
Ms. Shelia McCullough.

CONTENTS

PREFACE

What are your life goals? I encourage you to think about it for a minute. You are never too old to consider, "What do you want to be when you grow up?" That is as long as you do not think that you're too old to grow. Surely, you are striving to be a better version of yourself in some aspect of your life. So, what is it? Grab a pen and notebook, or use your cell phone, and notate some things that you would like to improve in your life. We are sophisticated people with multifaceted lives, and we have a multitude of dreams and desires. In other words, we are people with vision. We have visions of career success, attainment of wealth, family goals, dream vacations, and whatever else there is to want and strive for. We categorize our wants and needs on a hierarchy of importance and work to achieve and sustain each level.

The ultimate goal in life is complete wellness. Complete wellness is not just the absence of illnesses; it is much more than that. Complete wellness is the pursuit and attainment of physical, mental, social, spiritual, occupational, intellectual, emotional, and environmental well-being. Each element of wellness is like a cell in the body. The way we live influences the condition of the cells. We all would like to reach and live out our full potential, wouldn't we? As you aim to fulfill your aspirations and meet or exceed your expectations, how often do you consider your health? Did you include improving your health on your list of things you would like to change for the better? Why (not)? Maybe you added that you would like to lose weight. However, it is important to understand that health is not weight loss. Although losing weight can improve your health, many people who become ill first notice they are sick because they lose a substantial amount of weight.

Health is a condition of living. We can live in good or bad health. The conditions are dependent on our lifestyle choices. When health is called to mind, many of us think that we are okay. We assume this because we base our thoughts on how we feel. Instead, we should be looking at how we live and eat. We eat too much garbage, drink too much poison, smoke cigarettes, and overuse prescription drugs. But we feel fine. Our bodies can withstand some harsh treatment, but it doesn't mean that we should not be practicing healthcare as opposed to reacting to sick-care. Real health-care is preventative maintenance for the body. Sick-care is reactive - as we respond to symptoms of illness.

My purpose for writing this book is to share accumulated facts (knowledge) about health and clear up many misconceptions concerning diet-ing. I have researched multiple scholarly articles on diet, nutrition, health, and wellness. I use sci-ence and research throughout this book to sup-port my arguments and to add authority and cred-ibility to the discussion.

Dieting is a proven way to fail at weight loss. Dieting is an endless cycle of counting calories, re-stricting carbs, buying into weight loss programs, taking supplements, and obsessing over weight. The irony of dieting is that it causes weight gain. It is estimated that 80 – 95% of diets fail. While the percent range is not conclusive, it represents the reality that dieting ultimately fails. I think that is because diets are advertised and sold as a means to an end. Dieting is a tool to help com-plete a project – the project is losing weight. After the project is complete, the tool goes into the toolbox. And we do not adequately maintain the project.

The way you eat right now may not mean that much to you. You eat to satisfy your hunger – or to fulfill your desire to eat – then continue with a task until the next food break. However, your food choices are priming you for how you will look and feel years down the road. If you want to look good and feel good, you have to eat for the future today. To eat unhealthy is to be unhealthy. The opposite is true as well – to eat healthy is to be healthy. Instead of following strict weight loss rules that you will not maintain, focus on improving your health. People who live healthy lives are not motivated by weight. They are driven by being well, and they make food and lifestyle choices that reinforce their well-being.

I dieted for many years. I have tried different weight loss and workout programs, and I failed at each one – or each one failed me. I suspect that I failed for the same reasons that many others who attempt to "go on a diet" fail. I wanted instant gratification. Instant gratification is what is being sold to us in every bottle of diet pills, cases of slimming drinks, and weight loss programs. I had an idea of how I wanted to look, and when the weight loss programs failed to produce my expectations within an unrealistic timeframe, I would quit. I invested in miracle pills and magic potions that came short of promising results. I might have vainly continued down the path of dieting if it was not for my mom having a stroke. Although it did not kill her, it took her life – the life she used to live.

Her stroke put me on high alert. I became increasingly concerned about my health and well-being. I was nearly 100 pounds overweight, and my blood pressure fluctuated between stage 1 and stage 2 hypertension. Looking back on it, I realize that my food and lifestyle choices were the active ingredients which caused me to be a potential stroke victim. I stopped buying into the dieting gimmicks and started delving into health and wellness. I spent much of my free time researching health and wellness in every aspect. I consider myself to be a survivor - not a survivor of a medically diagnosed disease but a survivor of an unhealthy lifestyle that could have certainly caused some pernicious or sudden health complications.

Throughout my life, I have known many people – family, friends, and acquaintances – who have experienced the scare of a heart attack or stroke. Several of them were given second chances, but many of them died. Since the time of my mom's stroke, I have had more family, friends, and acquaintances who have suffered from heart attacks, strokes, and other health complications. I continuously hear people reason that they are experiencing health problems because those conditions run in their family. I used to accept this as a rational explanation, but as my knowledge of health continued to mature, I comprehended the relationship between food and life. It can be a toxic relationship, or it can be a healthy relationship. The choice is yours. I hope this book helps you to develop or reinforce your own health and wellness journey.

START OF A JOURNEY

O bese! That is what the results of my biometric screening made clear to me in October 2013. My body mass index (BMI) was 34. A healthy BMI is between the ranges 18.5 and 24.9. BMI ranging between 25 and 29.9 is classified as overweight. 30 and above is obese. Starting at the overweight range, the risk for health illnesses such as heart disease, stroke, and diabetes increases. I had been overweight nearly all of my life, so the results weren't much of a wakeup call. If anything, it only confirmed what I already knew. I was fat, or overweight, to put it gently. If I had taken the time to study the results, I would have realized that I was un-healthy. Nearly all my results were alerting me that I needed to make a change. I was ignorant to the fact that my diet and lifestyle choices were nearing me to the edge of several life-threatening medical conditions. My diet, which mostly consisted of fried and starchy foods, sugary drinks and alcohol, could have caused me to develop diabetes, high blood pressure, heart disease, liver complications, or some other life-threatening medical condition. I was not mindful enough to really understand the potential war that I was waging against my body. I saw my struggle solely as a weight issue. It had never occurred to me that my diet and weight were, in fact, health issues.

I was "husky" as a child. I lost weight during my late teens and subsequently gained it back during my early 20s. During my childhood, I did not understand why I was overweight. I was as active as the other kids whom I grew up with. We would run around and play seemingly all day, yet I was one of the two overweight kids of the group. I ate the same foods as everyone else. When grandma prepared her world-class fried chicken – *that's what everyone says about their grandma's cooking, right* – with mashed potatoes topped with gravy, green beans seasoned with pork fat, and served with cornbread and lots of love, we considered that to be a healthy meal. That was hearty food, soul food, country cooking. Meals like this were a staple in grandma's kitchen. The entire family ate that way, yet I was the only one who was overweight. Well, I was also the only one who went back for seconds and sneaked in thirds when no one was looking.

In addition to tiptoeing back into the kitchen for extra helpings, I would hide snacks in various places around the house and eat them when the coast was clear. Although I did those things and had some idea that my excessive snacking was a contributing factor to my unhealthy childhood weight, I still thought that I had been unfairly selected to be a fat kid. I had one friend in my tight circle of friends and cousins that was overweight too. Everyone else was "normal." I thought I was meant to be big. I learned to see being overweight as my "natural body type," but I was not comfortable with it. To make me feel better about being overweight, my mom would tell me that I was "big-boned." "Big-boned? So, my bones are fat, mama?" I remember asking my mom once as she tried to help me feel better about my weight. Although my mom was loving and encouraging, other family members and friends were not so nice. They would call me names indicative of my weight. I had become so used to hearing a variety of name-calling that I did not find them too offensive. Even though I could tolerate the name-calling, I would have preferred not to be called any of those names. My mom would always offer some comforting words after someone referred to me as Fat Boy or some other fat slur. Once, she told me that if I were skinny, people would still have something to say. Nonetheless, it always reminded me that I did not like my body. I was uncomfortable, and even as a child, I would make subtle efforts to lose weight.

The biggest problem that I had was one that many overweight people are faced with every day. I did not lack the desire to lose weight, but I lacked the know-how. I was clueless about how to get rid of the extra pounds. I did not understand the science behind diet nor nutrition, nor did any of my immediate family. I was often told that I did not exercise enough, although I rode my bike and played basketball with the neighboring kids nearly every day. Because I was a heavyweight kid, I was often asked – even by strangers, "Do you play football?"

> Me: *Shaking my head*, "No."

> Them: "Why not?" "You're too big not to be playing football."

Then, I am left with the embarrassment of being, as I often heard, "big for nothing." I was big for something. I was big because of my love for cakes, pies, doughnuts, cookies, banana pudding, peach cobbler.... you get the point. The name-calling would bother me enough to make me want to shed off some of the pounds. At times, I would feel guilty when I ate any of my favorite junk foods. I would tell myself, "after I eat this cookie, I'll start my diet tomorrow." Then, I would say, "since I'm waiting to start my diet tomorrow, I may as well eat my favorite snacks today." This was a 12-year-old me talking to myself like that. At such an early age, I had learned and begun practicing the unhealthy mindset of dieting.

Essentially, I was telling myself that I will binge eat today and start my diet tomorrow. I was eating foods at the moment to "get it out of my system." In reality, I was putting it into my system. This was a learned behavior. What would a 12-year-old know about going on a diet unless he was observing that behavior in his environment? I would snack throughout the day just because the food-like products were available. Food-like products? Yeah, manufactured products designed to look, smell, and taste like real food. The canned "food," SPAM, is an example of a food-like product. Velveeta "cheese" is a food-like product. Be honest, did you think Velveeta was real cheese? The eating habits that I struggled with during childhood followed me into adulthood. No surprises there.

I had become trapped in a matrix of unhealthy dieting and poor lifestyle choices. It was like I had been prescribed an endless refill of the blue pills because the red pills were hard to swallow. Take the blue pills and continue to live in ignorant bliss where you consider the knowledge of health as trivial information. Ignore the fact that food provides life, but it also causes death – often, a slow and progressively painful one. Take the red pills and embrace the knowledge of health. Learn the difference between proactive healthcare and reactive sick-care. Then, become disciplined and apply the appropriate methods to your life to benefit from a better quality of life.

It is difficult to eat to live when you have been living to eat all your life. If you are struggling with weight loss and find it challenging to manage a healthy weight, it could be because your concept of dieting is wrong. Ask yourself: "What do I normally eat each day?" You must consider everything – meals, snacks, and drinks. "How often do I eat?" Do you eat because you are hungry, or do you eat because "it's time to eat?" These questions must be answered honestly to begin to shift from a dieting mindset to a healthy mindset. A dieting mindset focuses on restricting food, losing weight, negative self-talk, comparing yourself to others, and not acknowledging your small wins. A healthy mindset focuses on eating to live, gaining wellness, positive self-talk, not being in competition with anyone, and long-term health.

By 2010, I weighed 230 pounds. That was not a healthy weight for me. I was not muscular nor in good shape. Nonetheless, I had gotten comfortable with being at that weight. As long as I stayed around 230 pounds, I allowed myself to think that I was healthy enough. My waistline was 40 inches. When I compare my photos from then and now, I look like a completely different person. In hindsight, it is easy to see why I was overweight. Look at a sample of my diet plan:

- Breakfast
    - 4 Waffles ~ 360 calories
    - with syrup ~ 210 calories
    - 4 scrambled eggs ~ 360 calories
    - 2 sausage patties ~ 180 calories
    - 20 oz. soda ~ 240 calories
- Mid-Morning Snack
    - 2 Doughnuts ~ 400 calories
- Lunch
    - Burger combo ~ 1,100 calories
    - Mid-Day Snack
    - Bag of chips ~ 260 calories
    - 16 oz. Energy drink ~ 200 calories
- Dinner
    - 3-piece fried chicken meal ~ 1,500 calories

I have provided only an estimate of my caloric intake in the example. I did not factor in the number of unhealthy fats and carbs that come with the type of foods that I regularly ate. I am sure the numbers are appalling. As I mentioned before, I ate throughout the day and was consuming nearly 5,000 calories per day. Calories alone were not my problem; it was the quality of the calories and a sedentary lifestyle. I had a high refined sugar and a fiber deficient diet. Refined sugar is why carbohydrates have a bad reputation, and my diet was loaded with that junk. Notice in the example of my diet plan that I did not eat any of the life-sustaining foods such as fresh fruits, vegetables, nuts, or seeds. I did not drink much water, either. I would guess that I drank about 50 ounces of water daily. While I did eat fruits and vegetables, I did not eat them often enough to be considered a part of my normal diet.

So, here I was, existing in a vitamin deficient, mineral deficient, and dehydrated state. I can only imagine the stress that I was putting on my body. My diet was full of saturated fats, simple carbs, and PROTEIN. Must have that protein, right? My thoughts about food were naive. I saw food as a substance to feed my appetite with all the things that I enjoyed eating. I did not view food as a source of fuel for sustaining life.

There were times when I would be overcome with a need to get fit. Whenever that happened, I would start following some fad diet and taking fat loss supplements so I could get the weight off. When reading up on those rapid weight loss diet plans, many of them recommended carb restriction or food restriction altogether. Through my hasty research, I was convinced that carbohydrates were the reason I was overweight. Because of the type of carbs I frequently ate, that idea was not entirely untrue. When reading a nutrition label, I counted carbs as though they were all the same. I did not understand the difference between simple and complex carbs at the time. I had become so used to hearing people swear by carb restriction that I took it to be the method for weight loss.

Anytime my weight range got about plus 5, I defaulted to a restricted carb diet. I thought of it as the method of controlling my weight. However, I was only trying to control a portion of something, whereas the whole thing was out of control. In addition to carb restriction, I would dust off my gym membership and start back exercising. I mostly focused on cardio workouts and divided my time between treadmills and ellipticals. Although I was making monthly payments for a gym membership, I was basically giving money away. I went to the gym periodically. In total, I may have gone enough to equal 3 out of the 12 months of a year.

I had always confused fitness and health. I used the words interchangeably and conflated them into one thought. I assumed that a physically fit person was healthy. My misconceptions about the meaning of physically fit were in terms of weighing a certain amount, having a lean or muscular build, or being able to bench press at least your own body weight. But I did not know that fitness and healthiness were not the same. As I became aware of proper dieting, nutrition, and the many concepts of health and wellness, I started to understand the difference between health and fitness. I also began recognizing the relationship between the two. I realized that both parts are essential to our whole well-being, yet they are separate systems that function within wellness. Nonetheless, some of the components from each system overlap, making health akin to fitness.

At the start of 2014, I weighed 250 pounds, and by the end of 2014, I weighed 190 pounds. I called it The 2014 Transformation. By making dietary changes over time, I dropped an additional 10 pounds. I have managed to keep the weight off by continuing to educate myself on diet, nutrition, health, and fitness. Reading books like *How to Eat to Live* by Elijah Muhammad and *The Mind-Gut Connection* by Emeran Mayer, MD, helped me become far more enlightened about the relationship between food and life. Watching health documentaries *like Fat, Sick, and Nearly Dead* and *Fed Up* helped me refocus and put health back as my primary goal. Before being introduced to those books and documentary genres, exercising and weight loss had become my motivation, but my journey did not start out that way. After I lost weight, I thought that I could eat what I wanted if I was doing fat burning exercises and maintaining a caloric deficit. My search for knowledge of health has helped me understand that we have the freedom to choose, or not choose, a healthy lifestyle. To be pro-health promotes a life of wellness as we remain attentive to our healthcare. To not select health is to select the sick-care system where we devalue the quality of our lives by continually making poor lifestyle choices and reacting to the consequences of our choices.

We frequently convince ourselves that family history is the cause of certain illnesses. Genetics makes us susceptible to developing certain diseases. Yes, it is true. What is also true is eating the foods that have made the family historically sick can cause the onset of the same illnesses and diseases in you. Here is an illustration of the benefits of making healthy diet and lifestyle changes:

Imagine that you come from a family where overweight and obesity are prevalent. Think of The Klumps from The Nutty Professor movies. You grow up not just eating unhealthy food but eating them every day with every meal - 3 to 4 meals per day. You do not give a second thought about what you are eating because it's "normal." Not surprisingly, you become overweight, and the weight gain gradually continues. Now, you are obese. Before you know it, health problems began to surface. You develop diabetes like grandma, dad, and aunties. Then, you are taking medication for high blood pressure like grandpa, mom, and uncles. There is a strange feeling happening in your chest area, but you are afraid to get it checked out by a doctor because you fear what he may say. At some point, you become sick and tired of being sick and tired, so you research, reach out, and renew. Research healthy diets and nutrition. Reach out to health and wellness coaches. Renew your perspective on health and work toward a healthy lifestyle. Essentially, you have embarked on a health and wellness journey. One year later, you have lost weight. The health complications are reduced or gone completely. You look healthier and younger, and you are no longer sick and tired. What changed? As you improved your diet and lifestyle, your health improved. Can you picture that?

The point I am making is an unhealthy diet should not be overlooked when determining the cause of sickly conditions. Illnesses may be genetically imposed to a degree, but diet and lifestyle choices raise or lower the likelihood of the disease manifesting. It is not so complicated. Family history puts us at risk for certain illnesses, but family habits decide the level of the risks.

Disclaimer - I am not a certified nutritionist, nor have I had any formal education in any medical, health, or fitness fields. However, I have learned many aspects of maintaining a healthy lifestyle through my own research. This book is not an attempt to provide medical, health, nor fitness advice. I encourage everyone to consult with your doctor and a certified nutritionist before starting any diet or exercise program. The purpose of

this book is to share my health and wellness journey and give some personal examples coupled
with scholarly reviews to show how a change in
mindset about health and wellness can lead to
reversing obesity and sickness. As with spiritual
journeys, when you start a health and wellness
journey, there is no end to it. If you are serious
about your journey, once you start, you will be
on that expedition throughout your life. I hope
this book inspires you to research, reach out, and
renew your knowledge of health and commit to
your own health and wellness journey.

READING THE LABELS

*"We are all warned to read labels. The salutary
truth is that we shouldn't be eating anything
that has a label on it!" — T.C. Fry*

The best foods - natural fruits and vegetables -
do not come with a nutritional label. Fresh produce, in its natural state, is good for us to eat. The
law requires processed foods to have a nutritional
label to show the serving size and the nutrient
contents of the food items. The importance of
reading the labels is to know what you are putting
into your body. Without knowing the nutritional
facts and ingredients in your food, it is like taking
medicine without reading the dosage or warning
label. Learning how to read a nutrition label is
fundamental. Understanding the contents of the
food helps us to make healthy choices. High blood
pressure and diabetes are created in the kitchen.
They say the same is true of abs. Eating a balanced

diet requires discipline. And it requires discipline to take a minute to read the nutrition labels.

We count calories to avoid overeating. We engage in calorie-burning exercises to get or stay fit. You have not done yourself any favors by finishing a high-intensity workout then eat a protein bar loaded with refined sugar. That goes against what you are trying to accomplish, assuming that being healthy and fit is what you are aiming for.

What is the meaning of fitness? Well, that depends on who you ask. The word fitness can be spread thin when it comes to defining what it is. Fitness can have a different meaning for different groups because it is activity-specific. Physical fitness for a powerlifter is not the same kind of fitness for a triathlete. In general, physical fitness is being able to apply the required strength and energy to complete specific physical activities. If a sprinter cannot complete a triathlon, then he would not be considered fit among a group of competing triathletes. Health is different from fitness, but like fitness, health can have several perspectives. In general, health is being free from illness and sustaining overall wellness. Health and fitness are often conflated because neither can be attained without proper nutrition. Nutrition information is a description of how you are either contributing to health and fitness, which are dimensions of wellness, or feeding into sickness and disease – dimensions of illness.

Before I began practicing healthy habits, I mostly ate what I wanted when I wanted, and my food choices were reckless. Today, I still eat what I want only with a completely different applied mindset and a far better understanding of nutrition. Before having knowledge of health, my focus was to maintain an unhealthy weight range that I had become comfortable with. When I was at my largest weight, I weighed 250 pounds. During that time, I could not seriously imagine being 180 pounds. My mindset was that weighing 180 pounds would make me look too small. This was an unhealthy mentality that was reinforced by my idea that health and fit where interchangeable thoughts. After I understood that what I was referring to as fit was actually health, it put into perspective that there is not a one-size-fits-all model. Healthy bodies come in different shapes and sizes. Although your weight alone is not a good measure of health, carrying excess fat around the waistline commonly is correlated to an increased risk of strokes, heart attacks, and other health problems.

When I initially started reading nutrition labels, I was only counting macronutrients. Macro is a prefix that derives from the Greek word "makros," meaning "large or long." Macro-nutrients are nutrients that are required in large amounts because they provide calories (or energy). Proteins, carbohydrates, and fats make up macronutrients. Even though I looked over how many grams or milligrams of each nutrient I was consuming, I really did not understand what I was measuring. As I glanced over a label, my mindset was all carbs are bad, the more protein, the better, and fat-free or reduced-fat was a preference. This was virtually my complete understanding of the information on a nutrition label. I thought of it all as trivial knowledge rather than how I was nourishing, or malnourishing, my body. I did not know how my intake of fats and cholesterol was really affecting my body. I knew that sodium was a cause of high blood pressure, but still, I did not factor how much sodium I was including into my diet. I was far over the daily recommendation of all the bad stuff and not consuming nearly enough of the good things.

Precisely what are calories? What is protein? What are fats? What is the difference between good and bad fats? What are carbohydrates? Are all carbs bad? If not, why are we encouraged to limit them by the fitness community? It is easy to be manipulated into thinking that you are eating healthy when, in fact, you are not. Many foods are advertised as though they support a healthy diet when they don't. Some food manufacturers will impress you with eye-catching packaging with **10 g PROTEIN** boldly etched on the wrappers. When you see this, flip it over and look at the nutrition facts. How many grams of sugar comes with that protein? How much fat? How much sodium? What is the serving size? This is why it's important to know how to read a nutrition label. When reading a nutrition label, start with serving size located at the top of the label and work your way down to the footnotes at the bottom of the label; then, read the ingredients. The following information is a brief overview of the substances that are found on nutritional labels.

Serving Size: The serving size information is located at the top of the label. Without knowing the serving size, it is easy to be fooled into thinking that the nutrition facts are in relation to the contents of an entire package. Instead, it is relative to only a portion of the pack. If a food item has 2 servings, then you would multiply the nutritional information by 2. Let's say that a pack of cookies has 6 cookies inside the wrapper. You notice that the package says, "only 4 g of sugar per serving." Not too bad, huh? So, now, you flip it over and read the nutritional label and realize that the package has 3 servings. That is, 2 cookies are 1 serving, 4 cookies are 2 servings, and 6 cookies are 3 servings. This means that by eating all 6 cookies, you have eaten 3 servings. Instead of the not so bad 4 grams of sugar, you have just eaten 12 grams of sugar – refined sugar.

Calories are units of energy. The more calories in your food, the more energy it provides to the body. Nuts are a healthy high-energy because they are calorie (energy) dense. 1 oz. of nuts is approximately 150 calories. Every part of the body uses the energy from calories to function. Calories are tricky because they are not the same. Healthy calories, like those you get from nuts, also comes with essential nutrients. High-calorie food products like candy bars are empty calories because they lack nutritional value. They are made of mostly refined sugar and carbs. There are 4 calories in each gram of carbohydrates and protein, and there are 9 calories in each gram of fat. Nuts are high in unsaturated fat, which explains why they are calorie-dense.

Fats help the body dissolve some vitamins, and they are vital for healthy skin. The body uses fats to store energy. Excessive storage of energy leads to unhealthy weight gain and health complications like the development of cardiovascular diseases. Fats are high in calories – even good fats – at 9 calories per gram. The different types of fats are

- saturated, unsaturated, polyunsaturated, mono-unsaturated, and trans fats.

  - **Trans fats** are artificial fats made from vegetable oils through a process called partial hydrogenation. This is the worse form of fat. It is so bad that the FDA has prohibited restaurants and grocers from using them. Natural trans fats are found in meat and dairy products. Whether they are artificial or natural, trans fats are harmful to our health because they lower good cholesterol and raise bad cholesterol. A surplus of trans fat in our diets can cause conditions like heart disease, stroke, or diabetes. Foods like movie-theater butter, vegetable shortening, biscuits, doughnuts, and other baked goods and fried foods contain small amounts of trans fat per serving. The nutritional label may show 0 grams of trans fat if there are less than .5 grams per serving. If the food contents have a small serving size, there could be a few grams of trans fat hidden in the food. If you buy a frozen pizza, and there are .4 grams of trans fat per serving, it will not be listed on the nutrition label. If the pizza has 8 servings, there are 3.2 grams of trans fat in that box of pizza. When referring to the list of ingredients located on the packaging, partially hydrogenated oils are the same as trans fats.

- **Saturated fats** are not as bad as trans fats, but that does not mean that they are good either. The American Heart Association recommends that you should "aim for a dietary pattern that achieves 5% to 6% of calories from saturated fat. For example, if you eat 2,000 calories a day, no more than 120 of them should come from saturated fat. That's about 13 grams of saturated fat per day." Saturated fats are saturated with hydrogen molecules, and they cause the fats to solidify at room temp. Think about how the grease (fat) from meat hardens after it has been stored at room temp after several hours. Red meat and cheese are high in saturated fat. There is another food product that is marketed as healthy, but it's not as good as advertisers claim it to be. Coconut oil has about 12 grams of saturated fat per serving. One serving is 1 tablespoon.

- **Unsaturated fats** are the healthiest form of fats. They remain in the form of liquid when stored at room temp. Unsaturated fats are commonly referred to as oils – like vegetable oils. They can reverse the effects of trans fats by lowering bad cholesterol. There are 2 types of unsaturated fats - polyunsaturated and monounsaturated.

- **Monounsaturated fats:** According to Harvard Health Publishing, "Monounsaturated fats have a single carbon-to-carbon double bond. The result is that it has two fewer hydrogen atoms than a saturated fat and a bend at the double bond. This structure keeps monounsaturated fats liquid at room temperature. Good sources of monounsaturated fats are olive oil, peanut oil, canola oil, avocados, and most nuts, as well as high-oleic safflower and sunflower oils."
- **Polyunsaturated fats:** Harvard Health Publishing notes, "Polyunsaturated fats are essential fats. That means they are required for normal body functions, but your body cannot make them. So, you must get them from food. A polyunsaturated fat has two or more double bonds in its carbon chain." Polyunsaturated fats include omega 3 and 6 fatty acids. Examples of omega 3s are fatty fish like salmon and sardines. They also include seeds and nuts such as flaxseed and walnuts. Examples of omega 6s are grape seed oil, sunflower oil, and olive oil.

Cholesterol is a fatty, waxy substance found in the body. The liver produces enough cholesterol that we need for proper body functions. Cholesterol alone is not bad for us; we need it, but too much of it has adverse effects on our health. Unhealthy eating habits are one of the common causes of high cholesterol. As cholesterol moves through the bloodstream, it can stick to the artery walls and begin building plaque. Over the years of buildup, the artery-clogging can get worse and cause a heart attack or stroke. Like fats, there is good and bad cholesterol. The good cholesterol is known as HDL (high-density lipoprotein). HDL cholesterol helps displace bad cholesterol. Bad cholesterol is known as LDL (low-density lipoproteins). HDL carries cholesterol from the body to the liver. The liver breaks it down in to waste and rids it from the body. Therefore, it is thought to be good. LDL is considered bad cholesterol. LDL takes cholesterol from the liver to the bloodstream. Too much of it causes plaque buildup in the arteries.

Sodium is a necessary nutrient for the body to function properly. It helps balance fluids in your body, transmit nerve impulses, and causes muscle contractions. However, too much sodium elevates blood pressure and increases the risk of cardiovascular diseases. We should avoid excess intake of sodium. The American Heart Association recommends no more than 2,300 milligrams (mg) a day. America's favorite restaurant, McDonald's, reports on their website that the Big Breakfast meal has 1490mg of sodium. This one meal constitutes over half of the daily recommended intake.

Carbohydrates are a primary source of food and the body's preferred source of fuel. There are 3 parts to carbohydrates – fiber, starches, and sugar. The body converts carbohydrates into energy more readily than it can fat or protein. Once digested, the starches and sugar parts of carbohydrates are converted into glucose. Glucose fuels the cells in the body to produce the energy needed for cellular functions. There are two types of carbs - simple and complex carbohydrates.

> - **Complex Carbs** are high in fiber. They are plant-based foods like brown rice, whole wheat bread, and beans. Eating these types of foods can support healthy digestion and maintain healthy cholesterol levels. When digesting complex carbs, glucose is released slowly into the bloodstream as opposed to a rapid sugar spike. The results of a sudden increase in blood

sugar is a sugar crash caused by simple carbs. Complex carbs aid in boosting the body's metabolism, burning fat, and reducing hunger. They support weight loss, so, instead of avoiding carbs to lose weight, you should eat the nutrient-loaded complex carbs to aid in weight loss.

- **Simple Carbs** are mainly already digested. Like fractions, simple carbs are broken down to their simplest form. The body does not have to work as hard to digest simple carbs because the carbs are in their "simple" form. As a result, it absorbs into the bloodstream quickly, causing a sudden increase in blood glucose. While fruit contains simple carbs, they are in the form of natural sugar rather than processed sugar. Fruit also has fiber and minerals, whereas a slice of cake, made with processed sugar, does not. Simple carbs are not only the commonly known unhealthy foods like candy, soda, table sugar, and pastries. They also include foods such as white rice, white bread, foods made with white flour, and many of the breakfast cereals that are marketed to children. Diets with a high intake of simple carbs can increase the risk of developing type 2 diabetes and obesity.

Fiber or dietary fiber is a complex carb that is added to the total amount of carbohydrates in food. It is the portion of plant foods that the body is unable to digest. Fiber is found in all plant foods; this is one reason why a plant-based diet is part of a healthy lifestyle. Fiber cannot be broken down into glucose during the digestion phase. Because digestive enzymes cannot break down fiber, it passes to the colon intact. A fiber-rich diet helps maintain regular and healthy bowel movements. It aids in controlling blood sugar, cholesterol, and weight management. A regular intake of fiber supports the fight against cancer and cardiovascular diseases. Fiber comes in two forms, soluble and insoluble. When reading the nutritional label, to get the net amount of carbs in a food, subtract the grams of fiber from the total number of carbs.

Example: 25 g of carbs

<u>– 8 g of fiber</u>

17 net carbs

- **Soluble Fiber** absorbs water to form a thick gel-like substance inside the digestive system. As it moves from the stomach to the colon, it attaches to cholesterol, sugar, and other substances to slow down their absorption into the bloodstream and to expel them from the body. This health benefit helps protect against the development of diabetes and heart disease. Oatmeal, beans, chia seeds are some of the foods that are rich in soluble fiber.

- **Insoluble Fiber** does not absorb water, so it cannot form into the gel-like substance like soluble fiber. Since it does not absorb nor is it dissolved during digestion, it speeds up the flow of substances as it passes through the digestive tract. It binds to water as it moves along, causing softening of stool and making it heavier – often referred to as bulk. The bulk from the insoluble fiber puts pressure on the colon to stimulate bowel movements. Some health benefits linked to insoluble fiber are the prevention of constipation and colon cancer.

Sugar is another carbohydrate. Ingredients ending in the suffix –ose are the chemical names of sugar. Glucose, fructose, and sucralose are some of the familiar ones, but sugar has several different names. Among the more than 50 names for sugar, dextrose, brown rice syrup, and malt syrup are some of the ambiguous terms. Sugar is not just found in cookies and pastries. Added sugars are hidden in so-called healthy snacks. Try to keep the servings of added sugar low in your diet.

Ingredients: The contents of the ingredients start with the labeling on the front of the package. Whole Grain. Whole Wheat. No High Fructose Corn Syrup. Source of Fiber. No Salt Added. When we see these phrases on the front of packages, we add it to the shopping cart because we believe – or have been misled to believing - they are healthy for us. Because manufacturers can be deceptive about what is in their product, ignore the healthy suggestions on the front, and read the actual ingredients on the back. Product ingredients are listed in order of quantity.

When looking at the ingredients, take notice of what I call the **Big 3**. The first three ingredients make up the largest amount of the product. If the first ingredients include refined or enriched grains, sugar, or hydrogenated oils, put it back on the shelf because it's not supportive of a healthy diet. You should think of foods with a long list of ingredients in the same way. Food manufacturers commonly add different ingredients of the same substance. In any food product, there can be two or three ingredients for added sugar. For instance, you may see high fructose corn syrup on the list of ingredients, and as you continue down the list, you notice molasses is on there too.

   I have always heard people say that they do not eat everybody's cooking. It is mostly due to the uncertainty of the cleanliness of the cook and their choice of ingredients. Ok, but you will eat anybody's cooking. What do you think you are doing when you dine out? The cleanliness of the cook in a restaurant lies in the integrity of the business. The same is true of their ingredients. It is as important to know what you are buying from a restaurant as it is from the grocery store. Do not stop at reading the labels on the foods you buy from the stores. Get online and read the nutrition facts from your favorite restaurants before you eat there again. You can also download nutrition apps to your phone that will provide information about your meal selection.

THE SILENT KILLER

"People with high blood pressure, diabetes - those are conditions brought about by life style. If you change the life style, those conditions will leave." - **Dick Gregory**

"High blood pressure runs in my family." How many times have you or someone you know spoken those words? I must admit that I now cringe when I hear people say that. Although I too once claimed it to be a fact, I now understand that developing high blood pressure – or any disease – is more complicated than simply "running in the family." High blood pressure itself is not hereditary, but genetics can play a role in our susceptibility to develop it. More importantly, when we share the same diets and unhealthy lifestyle choices as family members who have this condition, the risk for high blood pressure increases.

During my annual physical checkups, the doctor would make a note of my elevated blood pressure. Still, I did not pay much attention to it. In 2012, my blood pressure measurements were 144/93. That is stage 2 high blood pressure. The checkup in 2013 revealed 131/85 results – stage 1 high blood pressure. 2014's results were better at 129/72, just inside the elevated range. 2014 is also when I started my health transition and began my health journey. But in 2015, although I managed to keep the weight off, I reverted to a junk diet. The consequences of my diet proved to be hurtful. My top number shot back up to 144 while my bottom number stayed low at 69 – stage 2 high blood pressure. From 2016 – 2019, my results shifted within the elevated range. 129/70 in 2016. 126/75 in 2017. 127/79 in 2018. 128/77 in 2019. As I continue to improve my diet, I expect my top number to continue to decrease.

Through observation, I learned that there is nothing you can do to protect yourself from high blood pressure. It was just a thing that happens to you around a certain age because of genetics. Go to the doctor, take your medicine, and all should be fine. No one had ever mentioned – not even the doctor - how changing your diet or exercising can help control high blood pressure, so how was I to know? At a young age, I anticipated being on prescription medication for high blood pressure by the age of 40. When that time came, the medicine would fix me. Do you see the problem with this?

The correct thought process would have been to protect my health now, so I do not have to depend on prescription medicine later. I was throwing my health in the garbage with a poor diet. In hindsight, it is bothersome how I just accepted assumptions that were spoken as facts.

What is more bothersome is that many others have the same thoughts on health and wellness that I had. They have accepted health ailments because their medicine can treat – not cure - the problem. My frustration with that mindset is 1) it causes the development of an indolent attitude toward health because medicine is available to mask health complications. 2) Medicine alone does not eradicate health problems. Medicine manages the symptoms that are produced by the underlying causes of the illness.

I thought there was not anything I could do to prevent the onset of high blood pressure, so I did nothing. Many of my intermediate family members developed hypertension. Hypertension is the medical term that refers to high blood pressure. *Hyper-* means "excessive," and tension is to "stretch, strain." Together, hyper-tension is the excessive stretching and straining of artery walls by the extreme force of blood. No one seemed to be overly concerned about it, so I did not see high blood pressure as a life-threatening illness. I expected to live a healthy life as long as I saw my doctor and took the prescribed medications. This was a weak outlook on life. My perception of health was entrapped in a vague and ostensible reality. Taking prescription medication is like putting a bandage over a wound. The bandage does not heal the injury; it covers, or mask, the wound. Under the right conditions, the body heals itself. Healthy lifestyle habits, like fasting, and nurturing the body with nutritional food is the real medicine the body needs to heal. Hence the saying, *food is medicine*.

With sufficient knowledge of health, we will choose to live healthy rather than just surviving sickness. We have so much to live for. We should treat our diets and our bodies such as our will to live. My attitude about health and nutrition was not aligned with my desire to live. I would go out to eat and count calories, protein, and carbs by using a calorie counter app, but I never thought to notice how much sodium I was consuming or how much fiber I was not consuming. The first time I can remember paying attention to the milligrams of sodium in my meal disgusted me.

My wife and I were at one of our favorite restaurants, and after ordering our food, I began to log my meal in the nutrition app that I was using. As I logged in the creamy chicken pasta, my eyes widened with disbelief when I read 3,200 mg of sodium. The American Heart Association recommends "no more than 2,300 milligrams (mg) a day and moving toward an ideal limit of no more than 1,500 mg per day for most adults." Here, I was about to eat 3,200 mg in one meal. I recall being really disturbed by this. As I was coming into the knowledge of health, it was becoming increasingly hard for me to continue to eat food without considering what I was putting into my body. The more I learned about food, how it works inside the body, and the detriments or benefits of food choices, I began to see food as medicine or poison. This mental shift came about as a result of my mom experiencing the pain and suffering caused by a hemorrhagic stroke.

On Labor Day, 2013, my mom collapsed as she was about to go to bed. When I received the phone call, I could not believe it. I had just been with her a few hours earlier. My wife and I loaded our sleeping kids back into the car and made the 40-minute drive back to her house. I was frustrated because no one had called the paramedics. I called 9-1-1 as we rushed down the highway. I was quiet and reserved outwardly, but inside, I was a bundle of nerves. When we got to the house, the paramedics already had her on a gurney. They had her sitting up rather than stretched out, so I thought she was conscious. I got out of the car and made my way to the ambulance. I called out to her. "Mama!" I shouted out, but she did not answer. I got a little closer and yelled for her again. "Mama!" Still, no answer.

I felt frozen. It was like I could not move any closer. I watched helplessly as the paramedics lifted her into the ambulance. I saw her head fall into her chest and bobble. I looked to see if she was going to lift her head up, but she didn't. My wife and I drove to the hospital, and after a sleepless night in the hospital's waiting room, we learned that she had a hemorrhagic stroke. The doctor who operated on her came out to speak with us. He said that her blood pressure was 210/140. Numbers higher than 180/120 is falls into the blood pressure category *hypertensive crisis*. This means that immediate medical attention is required. The nonprofit academic healthcare organization, Cedars-Sinai, explains, "A hemorrhagic stroke occurs when blood from an artery suddenly begins bleeding into the brain. As a result, the part of the body controlled by the damaged area of the brain cannot work properly." My mom had a brain aneurysm in the thalamic region of her brain. One of her blood vessels ruptured and caused bleeding inside her brain. As blood leaked from the ruptured vessel, it affected other parts of her brain and caused severe damage.

I replayed the events of the day in my mind attempting to see what I had missed. I questioned how I could not have noticed that something was wrong. I remembered that she complained about feeling hot that day. She took a cold bath to cool off. She also stayed next to the air conditioning unit throughout the day. She was always complaining about being hot, so that behavior did not seem odd to me. In retrospect, I realized that hovering over an AC unit while sweating profusely was abnormal. Then, I started questioning why I did not have the awareness to notice that she was having a stroke.

Hypothalamus, Greek for "under chamber," is named because it is located beneath the thalamus (inner chamber). It plays a crucial in regulating body temperature, and the damage to that part of her brain was causing her to feel feverish. I later learned that she had fallen twice and seemed confused before going to her bedroom. The third fall was at her bedside as she was attempting to get into the bed. I know that if she had gotten into her bed that night, she would have died. My mom had prolonged, untreated high blood pressure. Although she knew she was dealing with hypertension, she was not making any of the necessary changes to reduce it. High blood pressure is dangerous, and it does lead to strokes. Some of the most common causes of high blood pressure are poor dieting with high sodium intake, excessive stress, and smoking. High blood pressure is known as a silent killer because while you may feel well, it is quietly causing severe damage to your organs.

The conditions that caused my mom to have a stroke were an unhealthy diet and stress. She added salt to nearly everything, even the sodium dense processed foods that she would eat. I was sure that her salt intake far exceed the daily recommended limit. She was also stressed. She told me of the frustration and disappointment with some of the circumstances that she was enduring. I believe her levels of stress had become chronic, and she was distressed. The American Psychological Association explained, "Stress is often described as a feeling of being overwhelmed, worried, or run-down. An extreme amount of stress can have health consequences and adversely affect the immune and cardiovascular [systems]. [U]ntreated chronic stress can result in serious health conditions, including anxiety, insomnia, muscle pain, and high blood pressure." Unhealthy stress levels are linked to high blood pressure. When we encounter stressful situations, our bodies release hormones that cause our blood vessels to become restricted and produce rapid heartbeats. In response to this, our blood pressure rises. This is the body's natural response. The problem is when the stressors are ongoing. In that case, our body is always tense, and there is an ever-present strain on the body. Now, our response to stress is unhealthy, and it can lead to an increased risk of high blood pressure, which can cause a stroke.

In 2013, the American Heart Association reported that 1 out of 3 adults in the US, age 20 and older, had high blood pressure. That is 77.9 million people. High blood pressure is one of the leading causes of strokes. The Center for Disease Control and Prevention reported, "Every year, more than 795,000 people in the United States have a stroke, [and] strokes kill about 140,000 Americans each year—that's 1 out of every 20 deaths." Statistically, in the US, people are dying from strokes at a rate of a person every 4 minutes. Although the stroke did not kill my mom, it ended her life. It ended the life that she used to live, and it ended my former life as well.

My mom is confined to a bed. She cannot walk nor talk. She is paralyzed on the left side of her body and has a restricted range of motion on her right side. Once a strong independent woman, she is now bedridden. She loved helping people and always put her own needs last. She was a family care advocate for the Caddo Parish head start program, and she took pride in being a service to others, especially young children. Today, she is conscious of the things around her, but her independence has been arrested by her illness. Two months after my mom suffered a stroke, her mom – my grandma - died. I was sad, angry, and at a loss. I took it hard but kept my feelings bottled up inside. I began to drink a lot more. I used alcohol as a sedative to calm my racing mind and help me relax. I went through a short period of depression. Not only was my physical health at risk, but so was my mental health. My faith, the support of my wife, and the start of my wellness journey helped me cope.

By the start of 2014, my health and fitness journey was underway. I am not sure that my reinvention would have taken place if my mom's health had not declined as rapidly as it did. I felt as though I had vicariously experienced what she was going through. In other words, I was able to see myself in her place, and it scared me. It made me afraid for my own health. One day, while thinking over what happened to my mom, I became curious about high blood pressure. What is high blood pressure? I felt like I should have known the answer. I mean, it is a common medical diagnosis, and I know so many people who have it. Just months earlier, I expected that I would develop high blood pressure, albeit I was already being affected by it. So, what is happening to the body when high blood pressure takes effect? In the article *What is High Blood Pressure,* The American Heart Association explains, "high blood pressure is when the force against the artery walls is consistently too high. The primary way that high blood pressure impacts harm is by increasing the workload of the heart and blood vessels — making them work harder and less efficiently. Over time, the force and friction of high blood pressure damages the delicate tissues inside the arteries." It is vital to keep blood pressure in a healthy range, so you need to be aware of your numbers. Not knowing your numbers can be a matter of life and death.

120/80 is healthy blood pressure. The top number, 120, is called systolic pressure. Systolic pressure is the blood pressure on the artery walls as your heartbeats. The bottom number, 80, is called diastolic pressure, and it is the blood pressure in between beats when the heart relaxes. Blood pressure is measured in *millimeters of mercury* (mmHg). The higher these numbers are, the higher the risk of stroke, heart attack, heart disease, and even kidney failure. An unhealthy diet is a primary contributor to high blood pressure. Smoking and alcohol consumption also increase blood pressure. Psychological factors such as stress raise blood pressure as well.

While at work one day, I was stricken with a terrible headache. I did not have any pain medicine, so I went to the onsite occupational nurse to get something to relieve the pain. While I was there, the nurse insisted that I have my blood pressure taken. My blood pressure was 144/93 – stage 2 high blood pressure. The nurse considered sending me home but instead warned me of the danger that I could be in if I did not take care of my blood pressure.

After witnessing what my mom was going through, I decided that was it for me. I was not going to take any more chances with my health. At that moment, I made up my mind to officially start my wellness journey. Before bed that night, I set my alarm for 3:30 AM – one hour earlier than I usually set it for - to give me time to go to the gym before going to work. I woke up suddenly when my alarm sounded. I remember feeling different. It was a feeling that I can only describe as transformative because I knew that I was about to change my life.

I did not quite understand what all this life-changing venture was going to entail. I just knew that when God allowed me to wake that morning, it was a different me that awakened. My mind was different, my energy was heightened. It felt like the excitement you got as a kid on the first day of school. I was ready for my transformation. I was operating from fear and excitement. My blood pressure numbers shook me up; I was scared for my health and wellbeing. But I was also excited about making a change. I went to the gym that morning before work and completed an hour of cardio.

We often take our body's ability to function properly for granted because we do not think of what life would be like if we suddenly could not walk or talk. What if you had a stroke and lost the ability to use one side of your body – or both? What would you do? What could you do? While writing this book, one of my best friends had a stroke. Before leaving work, he was having a conversation with a coworker. He noticed that he was having a hard time pronouncing his words. He rationalized it as being hot and dehydrated. As he tried to get into his truck, he could not lift his legs high enough to climb in. After throwing himself in the truck, he called his wife as he drove himself home. By the time he got home, the right side of his face was numb. He had trouble walking, and his speech was slurred. His wife rushed him to the hospital. Upon being examined by doctors, it was revealed that he had an ischemic stroke. An ischemic stroke is caused when a blood clot forms and restricts blood from flowing to a part of the brain. He has a long road to recovery. Now, he will need to start his own wellness journey to protect his health and improve the quality of his life.

Life is a gift from God, and we are given our bodies to house our souls. He created our physical and spiritual essence to be in unity – to serve as an interconnected oneness like the universe. The physical (material) forms the body. The soul, spirit, and mind are made of the spiritual (immaterial). Together, the tangible and intangible aspects constitute the whole self. The body itself is only one entity of the collective whole. We are obligated to care for our physical selves by properly feeding and nurturing ourselves to keep the body well and healthy. The mind, soul, and spirit also need to be feed and nurtured properly for the attainment of complete wellness. Many people feed their minds with positive thoughts and affirmations to cultivate a healthy mental diet. People align themselves spiritually through meditation, prayer, the study of scriptures, and fellowship. They practice gratitude, spend time in nature, and engage in different forms of worship to connect with the Most High God for a balanced spiritual diet. But when it comes to the body, people are neglectful. The effects of an unhealthy diet keep us from being balanced or in tune with the whole self.

The more conscious I become about the attributes of health, the more I strive to take better care of myself. My journey to health and wellness is all-inclusive. It incorporates physical, mental, and spiritual health. My spirituality has helped to improve my overall well-being. The contemplative practices that are associated with spirituality have taught me to look inward for self-reflection. Self-reflection heightens emotional intelligence and enhances knowledge of self. As we contend with the many challenges and vicissitudes of life, self-reflection is essential to gain insight and perspective of self. It helps us effectively deal with stress, reduces anxiety, and promotes growth. So, rather than irrational reactions to life's challenges, we can intelligently respond.

Stress is a part of life, but when we allow stress to become distress, it can make us more susceptible to diseases such as high blood pressure and a host of other health complications that are associated with it. Although dealing with stress can become a negative factor in life, does a bad diet have to be too? There are many health risks associated with unhealthy food choices. As a defense mechanism, we say, "We all have to die from something." Sure, we do, but why speed up the process or put our quality of life at risk. High blood pressure itself is not seen as life-threatening, so we have a careless attitude about it. Despite the severe health threats posed by high blood pressure, it often goes unnoticed, or in my mom's case, untreated. There are not any apparent symptoms. That is why it's called the silent killer. So, how do we overcome it? With a balanced diet. A real balanced diet is not fats, carbs, and protein. Instead, it is a healthy mind, body, soul, and spirit. Each element of self is crucial to the complete wellness of the whole self.

YOU ARE WHAT YOU EAT

"The food you eat can be either the safest and most powerful form of medicine or the slowest form of poison." -**Ann Wigmore**

So many people fall short of having good health because there is so much misinformation about diet and nutrition. Candy bars are cleverly disguised as healthy snacks, and fat-free foods are marketed as a healthier option. Foods labeled as fat-free may be void of fats, but they are often saturated with sugar and sodium. Even when you try to eat right, surprise! You are damned if you do and damned if you don't. I now understand why many of our ailments can be linked back to the way we eat. Diabetes, heart disease, high blood pressure, and obesity are each diet-related complications. If the diet is wrong, the health is bad. We must first learn how to eat to live, then apply that knowledge. I had to unlearn everything I thought I knew about diet, nutrition, and health. I had to reevaluate it all. Countless resources are available to help improve your knowledge of health, but it can be perplexing because one source of information contradicts the other, so which one is correct? Rather than becoming confused with an overload of information, I learned to focus on wellness and general health. This has been the focus of my health journey. I was afraid for my health, so my motivation did not come from wanting a particular physique or reaching a specific weight goal. I was motivated by wanting to live.

Diet, exercise, and weight loss all tie into health and wellness. By focusing only on losing weight, you may be tempted to try out a trendy diet or exercise regimen that is not possible to sustain. That means when you resume your normal eating and lifestyle habits, the weight comes back. The calories in-calories out formula do equate to weight loss; however, it is an oversimplified method. It is mathematically accurate, but it does not account for the quality of the foods you eat. If calories in – calories out were as exact as it sounds, the popular calorie counting weight loss programs would lead to long term weight loss and wellness. Exercise is necessary, and the types of workouts and the intensity of them depends on your specific weight and body goals. I prefer cardio – high-intensity interval training, jogging, jump roping, and stair climbing – because I enjoy doing it, and it makes working out enjoyable to me.

There are so many trendy diets with Atkins, Ketogenic, and Paleo being some of the most popular ones. What is a diet, though? Most of the time, we refer to diets as a temporary assignment. It is a thing that we do until we reach the desired weight goal. The Oxford dictionary lists two definitions for diet. The first definition is, "the kinds of food that a person, animal, or community habitually eats." This explains how we usually eat as part of our lifestyle. The foods and drinks that we consume regularly are our diets - such as a vegetarian diet, for example. The second definition is "a special course of food to which one restricts oneself, either to lose weight or for medical reasons." This definition is referring to dieting – such as going on a diet.

People go on diets, and some will lose weight. More often than not, though, when they stop following the fad diet, they regain the weight. Another word for fad is "trend." According to the Oxford dictionary, a trend is "a general direction in which something is developing or changing." The dictionary also states that a trend is "a fashion." So, when we conflate the ideas of a fad (or trend) and dieting, we come to realize that dieting is fashionable. People are sold on the latest diet craze just as they are influenced by the latest fashion trends. Today, it is a Whole 30 Diet. Tomorrow will be intermittent fasting. Next month, the trend will be an alkaline diet, then the Circadian Rhythm Diet. Finally, in the following months, we are back to our regular eating habits and wonder why we put the weight back on, or those ailments begin to resurface. It is because rather than following trends, we should be improving our dietary standards. A standard is the degree of quality. If we improve the quality of our diet and stick with it, we just may begin to reverse some of the sickly conditions that we are living with.

Before having knowledge of health, I yo-yo dieted for years. Yo-yo dieting or weight cycling is to continuously cycle between losing weight, regaining the weight, and dieting to lose the weight again. I would lose about 20 pounds and put it back on in a short time. I was taking diet pills, drinking diet soda, and following a version of a restricted carb diet. At the time, I did not realize the popularity of low-carb diets. It was suggested to me by a salesman at a supplement store. As I was purchasing my pills, he was directing me on how to take them. I remember he suggested that I limit the carbs and mostly eat meat and veggies. He gave me a sample diet plan, and I thought to myself, "I can do that." I should have taken the diet plan and left the pills. In hindsight, I wish I would have thought to do a web search on the prescribed diet. Maybe it would have opened my mind up about nutrition a lot sooner.

Furthermore, I wish I had thought to read up on the diet pills. If I had done so, I would have realized that the pills came with many harmful side effects and had terrible reviews. Nonetheless, I followed the diet plan and took the pills as directed. I lost some weight, and I attributed my weight loss to the pills, so I bought more. As I was working on the second bottle, I started to experience stomach pains. It got so bad that I had to stop taking them.

Shortly after, I went back to my regular eating habits and eventually gained the weight back. What if I had continued to follow the diet without the pills? It could have been a good starting point to get control of a healthy diet. I am not advocating low-carb diets, but when comparing them to my diet during that time in my life, any version of a restricted carb diet may have been a better choice. When I ate healthy, I looked and felt healthy. When I ate an unhealthy diet, I looked and felt unhealthy. I have the pictures to prove it.

We have all heard the saying, "you are what you

eat." Today, it is a famous nutritional proverb. The axiom suggests that our health is linked to the foods we choose to eat. It has been taken out of the context of its original meaning, however. The origin of the phrase "you are what you eat" begins with the 1825 publishing of the book The Physiology of Taste or Meditations on Transcendental Gastronomy written by a French native, Jean Anthelme Brillat-Savarin. The original quote reads, "tell me what you eat, and I will tell you what you are." The intent was to describe how geographical, cultural, and religious customs and practices influence the relationship between people and their food choices. Over time, we have abridged the original phrase and given it a new meaning.

What does "you are what you eat" mean today? Have you ever thought about the scientific explanation behind this saying? How do you become what you eat? Our bodies absorb the nutrients, and junk, from the food we eat and uses it as fuel for the body to function. The International Foundation for Gastrointestinal Disorders explains:

> When we eat such things as bread, meat, and vegetables, they are not in a form that the body can use as nourishment. Our food and drink must be changed into smaller molecules of nutrients before they can be

absorbed into the blood and carried to cells throughout the body. Digestion is the process by which food and drink are broken down into their smallest parts so that the body can use them to build and nourish cells and to provide energy (2019).

Scientists conclude that there are over 30 trillion cells in our bodies, and the cells use the nutrients to heal and rebuild the body. Each cell supports the maintenance and integrity of our body's functions. The small intestine absorbs most of the nutrients in the food we consume. As the nutrients enter the bloodstream, they are transported through the body by the circulatory system. The large intestines break down the remainder of the nutrients. The foods we eat determines the structure of our cells. Our cells are constantly multiplying and dying; we can lose and grow billions of cells per day. The cells are replenished by the food we eat, making the phrase "you are what you eat," a literal statement.

When we consume processed junk foods with little to no nutritional value, it is similar to putting bad gas in your car's gas tank. It may run for a while, but it will not be efficient, and eventually, it is going to break down and cost a lot of money to be repaired. The same reasoning can be applied to our health. If we saw our food as fuel for our bodies, maybe we would be more selective of the grade of fuel we use? When we first buy a new car, we put the best of everything in it. We get the high-octane gas and the best engine oil. We keep it clean and well maintained. We should treat our bodies as well or better than we treat our cars. When our diets consist of plant-based and whole foods, we will benefit from optimal cell reproduction. The foods we eat can either have an adverse or favorable effect on our cell reproduction.

Our cells make up every characteristic of our being, and it affects every aspect of our body's function. In the book *How the Cells Obtain Energy from Food*, Bruce Alberts explains the process of food metabolism. He states, "[C]ells require a constant supply of energy to generate and maintain the biological order that keeps them alive. This energy is derived from the chemical bond energy in food molecules, which thereby serve as fuel for cells. The proteins, lipids, and polysaccharides that make up most of the food we eat must be broken down into smaller molecules before our cells can use them —either as a source of energy or as building blocks for other molecules." During digestion, each nutrient is broken down to its simplest form to be absorbed by the body. Proteins are converted into "amino acids, polysaccharides into sugars, and fats into fatty acids and glycerol." As the food is metabolized, the body uses what it needs as energy. When you consume more calories than your body needs, both carbs and fats end up stored as excess fat throughout the body. Food that is not used or stored is expelled from the body.

Protein is made up of amino acids and is critical to the cell's structure, function, and regulation. The word protein originates from the Greek term *prōtos*, meaning "first." During early studies of protein, it was a theoretical idea that protein was the most essential or "the first quality" nutrient. Proteins do majority of the work in the structure and function of the cells. Our cells use the amino acids as building blocks for bones, muscles, cartilage, skin, and blood. We also need protein to produce enzymes. Enzymes are the catalyst to accelerate chemical reactions that happens within the cells. These reactions are necessary for life because they support many of our body's structures and functions.

Lipids are fats and oils, and the body stores them as energy. The primary function of lipids in our bodies is to provide energy for muscles and bodily processes such as our organs. Polysaccharides is a compound word. A compound word is the joining of two or more words. When combined, the words form a new meaning. Polysaccharides is a Greek term for "many sugars." Poly – many or much. Sacchar – sugar. They are carbohydrates, and their functions include energy storage and providing support to cells and tissues. Our bodies break down these macronutrients through the digestion process, and our cells use them according to their functional processes. Protein, fats, and carbohydrates are referred to as macronutrients because the body uses them in large quantities.

For about 9 months, I worked as a surveillance officer. It was a boring job. Shortly after starting, I developed a habit of eating a honey bun – the ones with white icing - a root beer and bag of chips every night. Making a vending machine run allowed me to break away from the monotony and walk around without actually taking a break. Every night, I ate those vending machine snacks in addition to the meal that I would eat during my lunch break. Once, while eating what had become my traditional vending machine snacks, my supervisor started talking about exercising. He was a short, thick-set guy whose favorite subject was about his "better years" referencing a time when he was younger and physically fit. He was going on about how he used to be in "top shape" and how many miles he used to run each day. He was giving advice on how to lose weight – a subject that he regularly advised on. One of my coworkers, an older man, slim with a medium frame scoffed as he bit into an apple.

The supervisor looked at him and said, "What, man?"

Coworker: "Maybe you should follow your own advice."

Supervisor: "Man, I can lose weight anytime I want to."

Coworker: laughing, "Yeah, right!"

Supervisor: "While you're laughing, don't you know that apples aren't good for you because they have too much sugar?"

Coworker: Scoffs "Now, I know you don't know how to lose weight because you don't know anything about food."

The conversation went on for another minute or so before they moved on. Over 10 years later, I had forgotten about the amusing conversation until one day, a guy questioned me about my diet. I mentioned that I ate quite a bit of fruit, and he began shaking his head in disagreement, saying that fruit had too much sugar and carbs. He was a carnivorous type. We debated on the subject and agreed to disagree. Although I vehemently contested his stance on overeating fruit, honestly, he had me second-guessing my thoughts. I was still early in my knowledge of health, and when someone challenged me on my mostly fruit diet, I would spend days researching over the details. "Can you eat too much fruit," I wondered. "Maybe I don't get enough protein," I thought. While searching for information to confirm what I had already suspected, I found several misleading articles suggesting that too much fruit can be unhealthy because the body is not capable of distinguishing natural sugar from refined sugar. On a molecular level, sugars are equivalent in and of themselves, but the nutritional value of sugars are unalike. Furthermore, it is not likely, or maybe even possible, to consume "too much" sugar from fruit.

Is it easier to eat a half dozen of doughnuts or a half dozen of apples in one sitting? Let's talk about it. Without any complicated explanation, you know that doughnuts are not healthy food. In fact, doughnuts are not real food. Instead, they are a delicious food-like product. To be considered food, it must provide nourishment to your body.

Conversely, you also know that apples are healthy, nourishing food. Your body knows this too. I like doughnuts, but I love my health more. It would be easier to eat a half dozen doughnuts rather than a half dozen apples. Maybe your food consciousness would prevent you from eating so many doughnuts. The doughnuts are simple carbs; there is no fiber, just fat and sugar. Without fiber, you are not going to feel full, so you will be able to eat more. However, your body will have adverse effects from eating so many doughnuts. Now, let us compare apples to doughnuts.

According to their website, a Krispy Kreme glazed doughnut has 10 grams of sugar. Nutritionix, a nutritional database, says that a medium-sized gala apple has 18 grams of sugar. Solely looking at the numbers, it would seem as though the doughnut would be a better choice based on the sugar content. Numbers do not lie, but they can be misleading. All sugar is not created equal, and our bodies respond differently when comparing how apples and doughnuts are digested. The sugar in apples is natural, and the apple has dietary fiber. As the apple goes through the digestion process, digestive enzymes break down the carbohydrate, and the liver filters out toxins like pesticides. Eat organic if possible. The toxins are expelled as waste and nutrients are absorbed to be utilized by the body. The fructose from the apple is stored in the liver and released over time which supports steady blood sugar levels. The skin on an apple is also loaded with nutrients. About half of the fiber in an apple is found in the skin. An apple has Vitamin C and Vitamin A. It also contains calcium, iron, and other minerals.

Now, let us look at the doughnut. The doughnut is made up of saturated fat and sugar. The
sugar in doughnuts is refined (processed) sugar,
and unlike natural sugar, refined sugar is not ac-
companied by fiber nor other health benefits. The
doughnut has 190 empty calories. Empty calories
are the calories from food that do not have any
nutritional value. When our bodies metabolize
doughnuts, the simple sugars are quickly digested
and absorbed in the bloodstream causing a spike
in blood sugar levels. The saturated and trans-
fats are converted into triglycerides. Triglycerides are the main form of body fat. The fats in
a doughnut cause an increase in bad cholesterol
(LDL). While an apple may have more sugar than a
doughnut, the way the body responds to each food
is entirely different. Just by looking at the grams
of carbs and sugar can be misleading. I like to say,
*"You can't just look at the nutritional label, you have
to look into it."* Knowledge of health is imperative
to the benefit of our overall wellness. Knowing
what we are putting in our bodies is part of the
battle against illness. We also have to be disciplined enough to make healthier choices. This is
definitely a sobering message because I still struggle at times with deciding to eat for taste or eat for
health.

FIT TO LIVE

"Don't Wait Until You're Dying to Think About Living." -
Kamilah Stevenson

Obesity is an epidemic. The addiction that the country has to the drugs we call food has swept across the nation. So, how can anyone become addicted to food? Here's some food for thought: In the article *Food addiction as a new piece of the obesity framework*, Jose Manuel Lerma-Cabrera, Francisca Carvajal, and Patricia Lopez-Legarrea explore the similarities between the theory of food addiction and drug abuse. They write:

> In recent years, there has been an increase in scientific evidence showing both neurobiological and behavioral relationships between drugs and food intake. Basic research using animal and human models has shown that certain foods, mainly highly palatable foods, have addictive properties. In addition, exposure to food and drugs of abuse have shown

similar responses in the dopaminergic
and opioid systems. These similarities
between food and drugs have given rise to
the hypothesis of food addiction (2015).

Compulsive overeating has resulted in more than just a growth spurt in our waistlines. Because of the excess fat, salt, and sugar in our American diets, larger pants sizes often come paired with increased health risks. The way we eat is a habit, and bad eating habits can cause us to take in an excessive number of calories throughout the day. It has the proven ability to lead to unhealthy weight gain. The Obesity Medicine Association defines obesity as "a chronic, relapsing, multifactorial, neurobehavioral disease, wherein an increase in body fat promotes adipose tissue dysfunction and abnormal fat mass physical forces, resulting in adverse metabolic, biomechanical, and psychosocial health consequences." The dictionary simplifies the definition of obesity as "the condition of being very fat or overweight." As someone who was considered obese, I was aware that needed to shed a few pounds. However, I never associated my weight with illnesses, nor did I think of my eating habits as food abuse.

With the availability of so many diet and fitness programs, it seems that there should be a program option to fit everyone's needs. Yet, obesity continues to rise. Why? Maybe it is because our expectation for weight loss results is similar to how we like our food – fast and convenient. I figure diets fail for one of two reasons: the results are not quick enough, or they are too fast. Allow me make it plain.

Typically, when people try to lose weight, they try out some diet programs. They are mindful of what they are eating, and they incorporate exercise in their routine. If they are not seeing results soon enough, they tend to abandon the diet, go back to living how they were prior, and continue to struggle with their weight. On the other hand, when people go on an extreme diet, also known as a rapid weight loss diet, weight loss occurs too fast. A combination of supplements, very low calories, and intense workouts melt off the extra fat. That lifestyle cannot be maintained. Over time, the extreme dieter realizes that those habits are unsustainable, and slowly but surely, they revert to their old ways. The idea is not just to lose weight but keep it off and be healthy.

Much of the controversy that surrounded the TV series *The Biggest Loser* highlights my point. There have been several *Biggest Loser* contestants to lose an extreme amount of weight during the show. Still, when they got back home, they eased back into their normal lifestyle, and slowly regained the weight – sometimes weighing more than they did before being contestants on the show. This is an example of why I believe to overcome obesity, health has to be the focus, not weight loss. There is no magic pill or potion to combat obesity. You only need the will to be healthy, then apply that will to transform your lifestyle. This is the fit to live mentality.

Imagine going to the doctor for a wellness screening. The doctor informs you that you have cancer. You will fight like hell to survive because you have the will to live. I believe that you should fight equally as hard to overcome obesity and the causes of it. The American College of Cardiology warns, "Obesity has consistently been associated with an increased risk for metabolic diseases and cardiovascular disease. An increase in body fat can directly contribute to heart disease." Did you know that health complications that can be linked to obesity and unhealthy diets are among the top causes of death?

The Center for Disease Control and Prevention reported, "Heart disease is the leading cause of death for both men and women. About 630,000 Americans die from heart disease each year—that's 1 in every 4 deaths." The National Cancer Institute figured that "in 2018, an estimated 609,640 people will die from the [burden of cancer]. The predicted cancer death rate dropped in 2019 with an estimate of 606,880 deaths." We view cancer as a potential death sentence because we understand the destruction that it causes on our health. However, obesity is seen as just a weight problem, although it is connected to heart disease and several other health complications. If people responded to obesity the same way they would react to cancer, I believe the overall health of the county would improve. You must take enough interest in your health to overcome or prevent illness.

You get out of health what you put in it. Disease in, disease out. Healthy in, healthy out. Look at the word *health.* At the root of *heal-th* is heal. According to the Online Etymology Dictionary, the Old English definition of heal is "wholeness, a being whole, sound or well." The Etymology Dictionary explains that *–th* is a "suffix forming nouns of action, state, or quality from verbs or adjectives." So, when we talk about health, we are talking about a condition of living. Health is the action we take to keep ourselves well or whole. Real health foods heal, and processed foods do the opposite which is to harm and cause disease. Merriam-Webster defines disease as "a condition of the living animal or plant body or of one of its parts that impairs normal functioning and is typically manifested by distinguishing signs and symptoms." Disease is a compound word. *Dis-ease*. Online Etymology Dictionary defines the prefix *dis-*, "word-forming element of Latin origin meaning 'Lack of, not' 2.' Opposite of, do the opposite of' 3. 'Apart, away.'"

The suffix *ease* is defined as, "' physical comfort, undisturbed state of the body; tranquility, peace of mind,' from Old French aise' comfort, pleasure, well-being; opportunity.'" When we put the words together, the natural meaning of dis-ease is "a lack of physical comfort," "the opposite of having a peace of mind," or "apart from comfort, pleasure, and well-being." Being overweight causes a lack of physical comfort. Sickness will cause you to not have peace of mind. Obesity keeps you apart from being well. Dis-ease is a lifestyle problem. A diet rich in processed foods, fast foods, refined sugars, salt, and saturated fat is killing us. To reverse the dis-ease, the plan is simple, but the path is not easy because it requires self-discipline. It requires gaining and applying a sufficient level of knowledge of health.

I yo-yo dieted and took weight loss pills for years because I was looking for a quick fix to shred to extra weight. This is what I have learned: **DIETS**

DO NOT WORK! Never go on a diet again. Going on a diet can be compared to a smoker who fails to quit smoking. First, you try to control your portions to reduce calories similar to a smoker cutting back from a pack a day to a half a pack a day. Next, you replace meals with supplements like protein shakes or meal bars – just as smokers replace cigarettes with nicotine patches and gum. Then, you find yourself fighting off cravings. You try to walk it off, drink water, and eat a meal replacement bar. It does not work. Then, you say, "I've been doing well; I can treat myself just once." Smokers, on the other hand, say, "I'm down to 5 cigarettes a day, I can go ahead and have an extra smoke this time." Finally, you find yourself right back where you started. The 15 pounds you lost are back – in the same way, 5 cigarettes turn to half a pack and then back to a pack a day.

If diets do not work, how do you lose weight? You must make lifestyle changes starting with your thoughts about food and health. Changing your habits is the fundamental key to successfully transforming your lifestyle. It can be a slow process, so you must set goals and deadlines. Without targets, you will likely procrastinate to the point that you will not achieve your goals. If you aim to accomplish them too fast, you may not be able to maintain and revert to your old habits. Some people can make rapid changes, like going cold turkey, but most people need to ease into the transition. Either way, the approach to creating a new you start with your mindset first.

Regarding mindset, Malcolm X stated, "Once you change your philosophy, you change your thought pattern. Once you change your thought pattern, you change your attitude. Once you change your attitude, it changes your behavior pattern. And then you go on into some action." If you change your thought process and learn to focus on health and not dieting, you will change your lifestyle to fit your new philosophy. You begin to reinvent yourself from a psychological aspect, and it will change your attitude about health and wellness, and it manifests through your actions.

By the end of 2014, I lost 60 pounds. I changed my lifestyle and some of my habits. I worked out nearly every day, counted calories, and took supplements too. After losing weight, I assumed that I could eat whatever I wanted to eat. My weight was at 190 pounds with a 33-inch waist – there was nothing you could me. I was back to eating my favorite vending machine snacks, but the difference was that I was extremely active and counting every calorie going in and out. I calculated my basal metabolic rate – the number of calories burned while at rest - and wore an activity watch to keep a count of how many total calories I burned during the day. I thought I had this thing figured out. Boy, I was wrong.

Even though I was tracking calories and maintaining a caloric deficit, I was eating junk. No nutritional value, no life-sustaining foods, no knowledge of health. I had forgotten my purpose. I started my health and wellness journey because I was afraid for my health after witnessing the ordeal my mom was going through. Now that the first number on the scale was a 1, I became more obsessed with my weight and failed to notice my health. All slim and fit people are not healthy. As I mentioned earlier, health is health and fitness is fitness. Each has its place in overall wellness, but they are not the same.

Many people - family, friends, and coworkers, had noticed my transformation, so they began inquiring about how I did it. I would often recommend different supplements and workout plans. I rarely mentioned food at all. I still had a lot to learn. I became obsessed with my weight and being a particular size, but I would soon be reminded that optimal health is **the** goal, not **a** goal. The word "*the*" is the definite article. The definite article specifies the noun or phrase. Therefore, *op-*

timal health is the goal, means that I am specifically trying to attain and maintain good health. Good health is the only goal just as *"the"* is the only definite article. Weight loss is *a* goal. *"A"* and *"an"* are indefinite articles. Indefinite articles identify non-specific nouns. So, *weight loss is a goal* means that weight loss is not the most critical focus but a part of a bigger picture. Having knowledge of health teaches that weight loss will be a benefit of good health. People will sacrifice their health to be a specific size. If you are in a healthy weight range, what good is it if you have an unhealthy diet?

When I went to my general wellness checkup in 2015, and the doctor told me that my blood pressure was in stage 1 hypertension, and my kidney function was "off." He reassured me that it was not a major health concern, but I should not ignore it. All I could say was, "damn." I looked good, I felt good, but that silent killer was working on me, and I was giving it the fuel it needed to destroy me. Ok, self, time to get it together. So, what is my next step? While trying to figure it out, I stumbled across Joe Cross' health documentary, *Fat, Sick & Nearly Dead.* It was the first of many motivating health documentaries that I found. I did not do a 60-day juice cleanse, but I did start juicing. I started searching for similar documentaries, and each one I watched helped me to change my perspective back to health and wellness. Then, I started reading. As they say, reading is fundamental. The first and most important health book I had ever read was *How to Eat to Live* by The Honorable Elijah Muhammad. I have not mastered eating only one meal a day, yet. Nonetheless, it was one of the books that helped me understand nutrition and how to eat to live.

Although I overcame obesity, my health was still at risk. Through reading books and watching documentaries, I was learning so much about health, nutrition, and wellness. I had become a student of health without enrolling in a signal college course on the subject. I had lost a significant amount of weight, but it was due to exercising and counting calories. I still was not eating healthy. My diet included a large portion of processed foods. Processed foods are manufactured for extended shelf life. Foods that are made for long shelf life reduces self-life. Diets high in processed foods lead to weight gain and obesity. Eating on the go, fast food, quick-fix meals in a box, sodas, and "fruit" punch are causing us to put on the pounds. Just look at the nutrition label on a bottle of "fruit" punch. It sounds oxymoronic because there is no nutrition in "fruit" punch, but there are about 60 grams of added sugar in a 20-ounce bottle.

Fast foods are so convenient that people tend to eat more of them. A high caloric intake, coupled with a sedentary lifestyle, equals weight gain. Weight gain leads to obesity, obesity leads to other health complications. There is a lot of information suggesting that a main factor of obesity is genetics. I am no scientist in any field of the study, but I must reject the notion that obesity is an inheritance. Sure, we have different body types, and genetics plays a role in our ability to burn calories and where we store fat, but this does not mean that our bloodline ordains us to be overweight. My common sense tells me if that were the case, people who are fat because of genetics could not lose weight. If you are genetically inclined to be obese, despite your best efforts, sorry about that, but you will forever be stuck in an unhealthy weight range. What do you think? Our psychological diet and physical diet are what conditions us to be fit or fat, healthy, or sick. That is to say, the way we think and the way we live determines our wellness. Both aspects are learned behaviors. We learn them early in life, and the concepts are manifested through our behaviors.

Obesity is not an adult disease. 1 in 6 children in the US is obese. In the medical review, *Obesity Facts in America,* Kimberly Holland points out, "Around 17 percent of American children ages 2 to 19 are obese. That is more than 12.7 million American children. One in 8 pre-schoolers is obese." I experienced childhood obesity. I weighed 190 pounds between the 8th and 9th grades, and my waistline was 36 inches. I was between 210 – 220 pounds in the 10th and 11th grades, and my waistline was 40 inches. By the end of my 12th-grade year, however, I was back at 190 pounds with a 36-inch waistline. The difference being that I was 7 inches taller.

There are a lot of fat jokes for fat kids. Some deal with it better than others, but it is physically and mentally unhealthy to be an obese child and adult for that matter. Childhood obesity can lead to low self-esteem and depression. Parents, I encourage you to get or keep yourselves healthy and instill that mindset and behaviors into your children. That is the *"survival of the fittest"* mindset. Although we associate the phrase with fitness and strength, it refers to the successful reproduction and survival of our offspring.

Childhood obesity is disturbing. The unhealthy diets – eating cereal with 12 grams of added sugar per serving or the McDonalds *Big Breakfast* with 18 grams of saturated fat and 1490 milligrams of sodium for breakfast – puts children at risk for life-threatening health complications like diabetes, high blood pressure and high cholesterol which leads to heart attacks and strokes. The American Heart Association reported, "The risk of stroke from birth through age 19 is nearly 5 per 100,000 children per year. In fact, stroke is among the top 12 causes of death for children between the ages of one and 19. Boys have a nearly 1.3-fold higher risk for stroke than girls. African American children are at twice the risk for stroke, and death from stroke, compared to Caucasian children." While the article does not mention diet as one of the causes of children having strokes, it does mention conditions that can be linked to a poor diet.

These conditions were once thought to be adult problems, but the children are not only eating the same foods as adults, in many cases, they are eating just as much of it. Feeding a child 3- or 4-times day with adult size portions ... for what? Leading this lifestyle, children who are obese will become obese adults. In the research article *Children's Report of Lifestyle Counseling Differs by BMI Status,* Stacey Kallem and others reasoned that "The rapid growth in childhood obesity may result in today's youth being the first generation in modern times not to outlive their parents." Eating to live is the mindset to develop and practice. Fat, sick, and nearly dead are the consequences of not doing so. This is a fact of life, and it does not discriminate on age.

The way we eat as a society is known as the Standard American Diet, and it is SAD indeed. The Department of Health and Human Services reported:

> Typical American diets exceed the recommended intake levels or limits in four categories: calories from solid fats and added sugars; refined grains; sodium; and saturated fat. Americans eat less than the recommended amounts of vegetables, fruits, whole-grains, dairy products, and oils. About 90% of Americans eat more sodium than is recommended for a healthy diet. Empty calories from added sugars and solid fats contribute to 40% of total daily calories for 2–18-year old and half of these empty calories come from six sources: soda, fruit drinks, dairy desserts, grain desserts, pizza, and whole milk (2017).

Eating those type of foods often are doubly SAD – Standard American Diet as well as Sick And Diseased.

Selecting convenience over nutrition causes us

to eat more of the empty calories that converts to fat buildup and sickness in our bodies. It is one thing to do it to our own selves, but to do it to the babies too is not fair to them. Get them off the processed foods and refined sugars. Encourage them to become more physically active. Although I was an overweight kid, I loved jumping on my trampoline, playing basketball, and bike riding. It was just fun for me. I did not see it as exercising. Each one of us is fit to live, but we have to get fit to live. Making lifestyle changes is hard, and sustaining them is harder. What is the alternative, though? Do not wait until you are faced with a health crisis before you care enough to live. We need food to survive, but our food cravings are detrimental to our health. A bandage will not heal the wounds caused by years of poor dieting. Only a lifestyle change can begin healing the sickness and restoring health.

THE SPIRIT OF FASTING

*"A diet may change the way you look, but a fast can change the way you see." - **Lisa Bevere***

One of the most cost-efficient ways for over-coming obesity and other illnesses is fasting. As I have said before, diets don't work, but fasting does. Fasting is a lifestyle, and it is as close to a magic potion as you can get in my opinion. Before reading books on health and nutrition, I was first introduced to fasting in the form of fasted cardio. I was following a fitness group on social media, and many people were posting about fasted cardio. I researched it to get a better understanding of what it was all about. Basically, when your body is not digesting food, you are in a fasted state. We are in one of two states – a fed state or a fasted state. A fed state is when our bodies are digesting food. Typically, it takes the body approximately 6 hours after your last meal to complete digestion. An example of fasted cardio is eating your last meal of the day at 7PM tonight, abstain from eating throughout the remainder of the night, complete a cardio session the following morning before eating anything.

Before applying fasted cardio to my lifestyle, I would often eat eggs and toast or a bowl of oatmeal before working out. It was challenging to go without food before engaging in high-intensity cardio because I was used to eating. However, I understood the science behind it, and I wanted to take advantage of the fat-burning benefits. When exercising in a fasted state, your body taps into its stored fat for an energy source. Exercising in a fed state will cause the body to rely more on the food you have recently consumed for energy instead of stored fat.

Fasting has gained popularity in recent years. Although it has gained much attention in the health and fitness community, fasting is not a new concept at all. Historically, fasting predates the famous Greek physician Hippocrates who prescribed fasting to heal the body. One of his famous quotes regarding health is, "The natural healing force within each one of us is the greatest force in getting well. Our food should be our medicine. Our medicine should be our food. But to eat when you are sick is to feed your sickness." The Greek philosopher Plato said, "I fast for greater physical and mental efficiency." According to the Ancient History Encyclopedia, before any of the Greek philosophers and scientists were advising on health and wellness, "Imhotep was practicing medicine and writing on the subject 2,200 years before Hippocrates, the Father of Modern Medicine was born." Imhotep was an Egyptian expert in many trades. His mastery of skills included science, math, and medicine. "He is the only Egyptian besides Amenhotep to be fully deified, becoming the god of wisdom and medicine." Encyclopedia Britannica points out that Imhotep "becoming known as a medical demigod only 100 years after his death are strong indications that he must have been a physician of considerable skill." The science and benefits of fasting have been understood and proven for thousands of years. The information is available for us to read, study, and learn. It requires discipline to apply the knowledge, but isn't your health worth it?

If fasting improves health, then it refutes the recommended practice of eating 3 to 6 meals a day for optimal health. In a scientific study, *Flipping the Metabolic Switch: Understanding and Applying the Health Benefits of Fasting,* Stephen Anton and others studied the metabolic benefits of fasting. The researchers explained that the "review is focused on the physiological responses of major organ systems to the onset of the metabolic switch: the point of negative energy balance at which liver glycogen stores are depleted and fatty acids are mobilized (typically beyond 12 hours after cessation of food intake)." The following paragraph is worthy of being quoted at length as Anton and others explain the positive impact that intermittent fasting has on the body in comparison to eating 3 or more meals a day:

Individuals with a typical Western eating pattern of three or more meals per day never flip the metabolic switch, and thus their ketone levels remain continuously low. Additionally, as their insulin resistance increases with excess weight and diabetes, the time it takes to flip the switch is prolonged. The different IF [intermittent fasting] eating patterns described in this article all flip the metabolic switch with varying frequencies and durations. Compared with an eating pattern in which food is consumed over long time intervals (typically 12 or more hours daily), IF [intermittent fasting] eating patterns may result in a wide range of beneficial effects on health, including improved glucose metabolism reduced inflammation, reduced blood pressure, improved cardiovascular health, and increased resistance of cells to stress and disease in humans. These effects have been clearly established in animal studies as described above, but only some of these adaptations to [intermittent fasting] have been investigated in humans, and then they are typically investigated in subjects who are overweight or have obesity (2018).

Another health benefit that intermittent fasting stimulates is autophagy.

In the medical review, *Autophagy: What You Need to Know,* Sara Lindberg explains, "Autophagy is the body's way of cleaning out damaged cells, in order to regenerate newer, healthier cells. 'Auto' means self and 'phagy' means eat. So, the literal meaning of autophagy is 'self-eating.' It's also referred to as 'self-devouring.'" Autophagy is a systematic self-cleaning process that is essential for protecting the body against the development of diseases.

Intermittent fasting is a lifestyle choice for me. There are alternative ways to intermittent fast, but I primarily practice the time-restricted fast using the 16/8 method. The 16/8 method is to eat within 8 hours and fast for 16 hours. Because I work rotating shifts and swap from days to nights, I adjust my 8-hour eating period to my work schedule. When I work during the day shifts,

I typically eat between 11 AM – 7 PM. On night shifts, I aim to eat between 2PM – 10 PM. During the 16 hours fast, I only drink spring or distilled water, unsweetened herbal teas, and black coffee. To break my fast, I eat fresh fruit or have a fruit smoothie. After fasting for several hours or days, you want to ease your body back into a fed state to avoid digestive discomforts like bloating. Breaking your fast is the intention behind the word "*breakfast*." Breakfast was not intended to be bacon and eggs. Instead, break-fast is supposed to be nutritional plant-based foods that eases your body back into a fed state.

Intermittent fasting focuses on when to eat rather than what to eat. Instead of thinking of fasting as food restriction, think of it as preventive maintenance for the body. Besides the 16/8 method, there are other ways to fast. There is the 5:2 fast and the complete 24 hours fast. On the 5:2 fast, you eat a sensible diet for 5 days of the week and restrict your calorie intake to 500 for the other 2 days. An example of this is having up to 2,000 calories per day from Saturday – Tuesday, eat up to 500 calories on Wednesday, eat sensibly on Thursday, and 500 calories on Friday. The 24 hours fast is completely abstaining from food for 2 or 3 select days per week. An example would be to eat your normal diet from Monday – Wednesday. If you eat dinner at 8 PM on Wednesday night, you will not eat again until 8 PM on Thursday. Then, follow this sequence for the rest of the week.

Other types of fasting include water fast, dry fast, and partial fast. As the name suggests, during a water fast, you only drink water for the duration of the fast. You do not drink coffee, tea, or other beverages while water fasting. There is not a specific timeframe for this fast, but a general rule of thumb is to water fast no more than 3 days at a time. Dry fasting is a fast that effectively involves zero intake of any foods or liquids for the duration of the fast. Perhaps the best examples of dry fasting are practiced during The Holy Month of Ramadan observed by Muslims and Yom Kippur – Day of Atonement – the solemn religious fast of the Jewish faith.

Ramadan is the holy month of fasting and self-restraint. During this time, Muslims dry fast from sunrise to sunset. The period of Yom Kippur is the annual Jewish observance of fasting, prayer, and repentance, which is practiced by 25 hours of dry fasting. One of the health concerns of dry fasting is dehydration, but when it is applied with proper guidance and understanding, the threat of dehydration is minimum. The two types of dry fasting are hard and soft dry fasts. A soft dry fast is one where you do not drink water, but you can use water for daily hygiene. In contrast, hard dry fasting is to resist all exposure to water for the period of the fast. Partial fasting is similar to cleansing or detoxing. It is a limited fast where you avoid specific foods for a prolonged period. Those 30-day challenges where you go without fried foods, chips, sodas, candy, etc. are examples of a partial fast.

Many people attempt fasting as a weight loss approach. While it can support shedding extra pounds, remember diets do not work. A temporary diet brings about temporary results. If you decide to intermittent fast as a way to go on a diet, after you choose to stop being disciplined enough to keep cycling between periods of eating and fasting, the weight will return. Further insult to the body is that the weight that is regained is generally all fat. Fasting should be implemented as a way of living. Critics claim that fasting is a starvation diet. Their sentiment is not based on a proper understanding, however.

Fasting, in general, is concerned with time restriction. Thus, it is the act of voluntarily abstaining from eating for a certain amount of time. On the contrary, starvation diets emphasize food restriction, and its method is synonymous with rapid weight loss diets. In any health and wellness journey, it is imperative that you do not allow the scale to become the center of your journey. It will cause you to sample many unfit diet plans and programs that only produce vain or superficial results. The results of a starvation diet are like hitting a large jackpot at a casino and playing all the winning back. Your winnings (in this case, the winnings are weight loss) dissipate in a short time for lack of discipline, knowledge of health, and the miseducation of dieting.

Although fasting has many physiological benefits, it is a way to renew one's spiritual wellness. Complete wellness is to be of sound mind, body, soul, and spirit. The physical discomfort of refraining from food is a small sacrifice in comparison to the spiritual reward of connecting with God. Examples of fasting can be found throughout the bible. Moses, Elijah, and Jesus each fasted for forty days and nights. Moses fasted for forty days and forty nights while he received The Ten Commandants on Mount Sinai (Exodus. 34:28, Deuteronomy 9:18). Elijah fasted forty days and forty nights while he fled to Mount Horeb – also known as Mount Sinai or The Mountain of God - (1 Kings 19:7-8). Jesus started preaching after fasting in the wilderness for forty days and nights (Matt. 4:1-11).

Spiritual fasting is more about feeding the spirit with the divine words of God than it is about denying the body of food. Focusing on God and denying yourself of food, alcohol, smokes, and any other vices are required to be considered a spiritual fast. Imagine having to walk around blindfolded for a day. If you cannot physically see, you must rely on your other senses to interpret your environment. Your sense of hearing and touch will heighten to help you navigate along. Fasting on spiritual principles is likened to the experience of walking around blindfolded. When you fast and direct your attention to God, it will enhance your spiritual growth with a determined focus to become enlightened and inspired by God's words.

After fasting for forty days and nights, the devil attempted to trick Jesus into turning stones to bread. In Matthew 4:4 (NIV) Jesus answered, "It is written: 'Man shall not live on bread alone, but on every word that comes from the mouth of God.'" Jesus was referencing Deuteronomy 8:3 (NIV) where Moses said, "He humbled you, causing you to hunger and then feeding you with manna, which neither you nor your ancestors had known, to teach you that man does not live on bread alone but on every word that comes from the mouth of the Lord." Although some may argue that fasting is not required of Christians, it is prescribed. During Jesus' Sermon on the Mount, he taught on how to conduct yourself "when," not if, you fast. Jesus said, "When you fast, do not look somber as the hypocrites do, for they disfigure their faces to show others they are fasting. Truly I tell you, they have received their reward in full. But when you fast, put oil on your head and wash your face, so that it will not be obvious to others that you are fasting, but only to your Father, who is unseen; and your Father, who sees what is done in secret, will reward you" (Matthew 6: 16-18,NIV). The act of fasting combined with prayer can permit us to gain divine wisdom and guidance. Fasting and praying are not fad approaches to spiritual discipline and should not be practiced based on popular culture. They are biblically based disciplines for a spiritual purpose. Fasting for health reasons has many proven benefits. However, fasting for spiritual reasons requires a different mindset. Faith-based fasting does not come from our own strength and will but from the strength and will of God.

In the bible, the book of Daniel makes two references to Daniel's diet that has inspired many people to practice it as a partial fast. The first mention of Daniel's diet is in Daniel 1. Daniel rejected food from the king's table because he did not want to "defile himself with the royal food and wine, and he asked the chief official for permission not to defile himself this way" (Daniel 1:8, NIV). The royal foods must have been foods that were not consistent with the Jewish dietary law. Daniel was a righteous Israelite and held fast to the laws. Daniel convinced the king's official to feed him and his companion's only vegetables and water for ten days, then compare their appearance to the other men who ate the royal foods. The official hesitantly agreed, and after ten days, Daniel and his companions appeared to be healthier and better nourished than the other men – *see bible verses Daniel 1:3-15*.

In Daniel 10:1-3 (NIV), the scriptures read, "In the third year of Cyrus king of Persia, a revelation was given to Daniel (who was called Belteshazzar). Its message was true, and it concerned a great war. The understanding of the message came to him in a vision. At that time, I, Daniel, mourned for three weeks. I ate no choice food; no meat or wine touched my lips; and I used no lotions at all until the three weeks were over." Both chapters, Daniel 1 and 10, describes what we would call a partial fast. Daniel and his companions abstained from the royal foods and ate a vegan diet in Daniel 1. Daniel 10 shows that he resigned himself to eating menial foods for three weeks.

People practice the Daniel fast for faith-based reasons, and it requires self-discipline to adhere to the fast. Whether you follow the Daniel fast for 10 or 21 days, the dietary rules are generally the same. The dietary practices of the Daniel fast are to eat a classic vegan diet; however, vegetables should be the basis of the diet. Fruit, whole grains, beans, nuts, and seeds should be eaten moderately. With a classic vegan diet, processed plant-based foods are excluded from the meal plan. Daniel did not eat plant-based "meat."

Researchers have conducted studies to examine the potential health effects of this particular fast. In the research article, *Effect of a 21-day Daniel Fast on metabolic and cardiovascular disease risk factors in men and women,* led by Richard Bloomer, the researchers had 43 participants follow a classic vegan diet for 21 days. At the end of the study, the researchers concluded, "Results from the present study indicate that a 21-day Daniel Fast 1) significantly reduces systolic and diastolic blood pressure, 2) significantly reduces total, LDL, and HDL cholesterol. This suggests that a wide variety of individuals may benefit from a dietary approach in accordance with the Daniel Fast." The research shows that science and scripture are aligned – as they should be – and following Daniel's diet leads to improved health.

In the Old Testament, the Jews fasted frequently. The metaphysical benefits of fasting are often disregarded today, but it should not be taken for granted that God's people saw the need to make fasting a routine practice. Fasting is not only an Old Testament custom. In the New Testament, there are accounts where believers practiced fasting. Consider the following scriptures from the Old and New Testaments for examples of fasting:

2 Samuel 1:12 (NIV) "They mourned and wept and fasted till evening for Saul and his son Jonathan, and for the army of the Lord and for the nation of Israel, because they had fallen by the sword."

Ezra 10:6 (NIV) "Then Ezra withdrew from before the house of God and went to the room of Jehohanan son of Eliashib. While he was there, he ate no food and drank no water, because he continued to mourn over the unfaithfulness of the exiles."

Joel 2:12 (NIV) ""Even now," declares the LORD, "return to me with all your heart, with fasting and weeping and mourning.""

Luke 2:36-37 (NIV) "And there was a prophetess, Anna, the daughter of Phanuel, of the tribe of Asher. She was advanced in years, having lived with her husband seven years from when she was a virgin, and then as a widow until she was eighty-four. She did not depart from the temple, worshiping with fasting and prayer night and day.

Acts 13: 2-3 (NIV) "While they were worshiping the Lord and fasting, the Holy Spirit said, 'Set apart for me Barnabas and Saul for the work to which I have called them. So, after they had fasted and prayed, they placed their hands on them and sent them off."

Fasting has its place for the betterment of the mind, body, soul, and spirit. Whether you engage in fasting for the physical health benefits or for spiritual growth – or both - it requires self-discipline. From a physical point of view, it renews your health and the conditions of the body. Spiritually, it is a way to recalibrate the spirit and reawaken the mind – the kind of mind that was in Christ Jesus (Philippians 2: 5). Spiritual fasting can be abused when it is done with a self-righteous mindset. Isaiah 58 rebukes shallow worshipers who glorify themselves through the act of fasting. Although they fasted, they still committed unrighteous deeds. Therefore, when they fasted, it was superficial - an insincere religious ritual.

FOOD FOR THOUGHT

*"Health isn't just what you're eating. It's what you're thinking and what you're saying." - **Unknown***

All of our actions begin with a thought. The way we think of ourselves and the world around us governs our attitude and behavior. Our thoughts, beliefs, and attitudes are the structure of our psychological diet. The way we think is just as important as the way we eat. The body becomes what the foods are just as the mind becomes what the thoughts are. Careless thoughts can be as damming to our health as mindless eating. We know that an unhealthy physical diet can cause diseases like cancer, diabetes, and high blood pressure. However, the effects of an unfit psychological diet are not so evident. Or is it?

Maybe, a malnourished psychological diet is apparent, but due to the lack of knowledge of health, we are attributing its effects to other causes. On the surface, poor health is connected to an unhealthy physical diet. If we dig a little deeper, then perhaps we would find that at the root of the adverse health conditions is a malnourished thought diet. Our food choices are the result of the way we think about diet and nutrition. Therefore, **the** (*definite article*) root cause of poor health starts with our thought processes. Our psychological diet is what has us overweight and sick. Our thoughts are manifested through our actions, so before our physical diets can become unhealthy, our concept of diet is flawed first.

"Change your mind, change your life" is a proverb that indicates the power of thought. Hmm, the power of thought. Just how powerful is thought? In the book, *Train Your Mind Change Your Brain*, author Sharon Begley reasons:

> The actions we take can literally expand or contract different regions of the brain. In response to actions and experiences of its owner, a brain foregoes stronger connections in circuits that underlie one behavior or thought and weakens connections in others. Most of this happens because of what we do and what we experience of the outside world. But there are hints that mind-sculpting can occur with no input from the outside world. That is,

the brain can change as a result of the thoughts we have thought. A few findings suggest that brain changes can be generated by pure mental activity: merely thinking about playing the piano leads to measurable, physical change in the bran's motor cortex, and thinking about thoughts in certain ways can restore mental health (2008).

Our perception of things is the reality that we experience. Our perception controls our perspective, and when we change our minds (perception), we change our outlook of life (perspective). This mental activity can influence a completely new way of life.

There is a sea of information being processed by our brains. Whether consciously or subconsciously, we process tens of thousands of thoughts each day. We respond so fast to our thoughts that the thought itself is not always obvious. Have you ever just blurted something out "without thinking" or responded to a situation so fast that "reflexes" took over? Well, it does not happen without the mind creating the thought, then the brain processing the information and commanding the action to be performed. The speed of light is 186,000 miles per second. At that speed, it takes 8 minutes for the light from the sun to reach the earth at 93, 000,000 miles away. The speed of sound is 1,120 feet per second. The earth rotates on its axis at 1,037 1/3 miles per hour. All of these measurements are remarkable, but are they as phenomenal as the speed at which we process and respond to thought?

The speed of thought is not easily measured. Due to its complexity, it can significantly vary on a timescale. We have intuitive thoughts that are based on our senses and feelings. Then, we have analytical thoughts that require logic and deliberate cognition. To attempt to quantify the speed of thought, we would need to know its beginning and end. Thought is an abstract in-trapersonal process. Although we share a collect-ive consciousness with social groups and society, our thoughts still take place within self. Through a complex network of electrical signals, the brain gives power to thought, but thought is not pro-duced by the brain. These electrical signals in-duce the mental commands that initiate physical responses. My cursory research on the speed of thought lead me to an interesting blog titled *How Fast is Your Brain* by Jeff Bollow. The article at-tempts to quantify how fast a thought is mani-fested into an action. He suggests that:

> The human brain has about 100 billion neurons, and each one fires (on average) about 200 times per second. And each

neuron connects to about 1,000 other neurons. Therefore, every time each neuron fires a signal, 1,000 other neurons get that information. When we do the math:

100 billion neurons

200 firings per second

x 1,000 connections

20,000,000,000,000,000 bits of info transmitted per second (2009).

That is 20 quadrillion. If the transmission of these impulses were any indication of the speed of thought, the measurements scientifically and mathematically confirm that we are God's best creation. If we are His best, then, why do we treat ourselves so bad? Not only do we have poor diets and unhealthy lifestyles, but we become defensive when our unhealthy way of life is challenged. We say, "My grandparents ate this way, and they lived to be 80 years old." I argue the difference between living to be 80 and being alive until 80. To be alive is to breathe. Living, on the other hand, is measured by the quality of one's life.

As humans, we have great brainpower. We are capable of thinking our way through any situation that we are faced with. We have knowledge of food, as in we have a general idea of which foods are healthy as opposed to which ones are unhealthy. Apples or doughnuts? Cashews or chips? Berries or ice cream? It is simple, right? However, we often starve our health to feed our taste buds. We do this not because of what we know about food but because of how we think about food. Having knowledge of something does us no good if we do not apply what we know. Knowing is half the battle, so what is the other half? I would suggest wisdom. Knowledge has the potential to be power. When you transfer knowledge into action, it becomes applied knowledge. Applied knowledge is wisdom, and wisdom is power. If we were wise about health and food, we would not be so out of shape, overweight, and sick because we would be acting on what we know.

The way we think about food is a learned characteristic of our psyche. As children, we eat what is on our plate. We eat what we are told to eat, but we also eat what we are allowed to eat. From the time I was a child up until recent years, I believed that food was just as much fried chicken, mashed potatoes with gravy, green beans seasoned with pork fat, and cornbread (the foods I was told to eat) as it was potato chips, candy bars, and pastries (the foods I was allowed to eat). I ate candy and cookies as often as I could. I was allowed to eat them. Other than a few cavities, what was the harm in eating refined sugar? I ate sausage patties for breakfast. I was told to eat them. I am not saying that I made any arguments about what I was told or allowed to eat. What was the problem with eating meat packed with sodium and saturated fat? The foods tasted good, but they did not provide any nutritional value. Eventually, we develop our own palates of food combinations and flavors based on how we have learned to eat. Once your palate has been established, it takes a determined will to acquire a new taste.

In a Psych Central article titled *The Psychology of Diets*, Jane Collingwood discusses the fact that food preferences are a result of learned behavior. Collingwood quotes psychologist, Dr. Jeff Brunstrom, "There is every indication that most of our flavor preferences and dietary behaviors are learned."

Collingwood continues, "[Brunstrom] explains that several types of dietary learning have been identified, such as linking flavors with other flavors, and associating flavors with bodily sensations like fullness. Some of these processes may take place outside awareness, he suggests, as a form of automatic learning. But being aware of our preferences and choices can help us alter learned patterns." How do you suppose that we alter learned patterns? To do so requires us to not just be aware, but we also must be willing.

Exercising the will to do something different is how learned patterns are altered. Let me be clear: I am not advocating a diet of bland, flavorless foods. However, I am in favor of choosing health first, then make the foods fit your preferred taste. Think about it, when you cook your meat, you add herbs and seasonings to it to make it taste more like what? To make it taste more like the plants you have added for flavor. Am I right?

I often find myself engaged in light-hearted debates regarding the way I eat or choose not to eat, rather. Even before I became a seafood-vegetarian (pescatarian), I began changing my old dietary habits. I stopped eating pork and refused to eat anything that had been cooked with pork. My new way of eating piqued many people's interest. I am from the south. Where I'm from, many people proudly boast that "every part of the pig is eaten except for the oink." So, my diet was odd to some and offensive to a few. You may be wondering how my diet could be offensive. What we choose to eat, or not eat, can spark as much debate as religion, politics, and sports. Do you find that hard to believe? Tell a vegan why you believe animal fats and protein from animal flesh are essential to our diets. Be prepared to argue. I caution you, though, because vegans will have science on their side.

Our thoughts and beliefs make up who we are. Because our identity is tangled up in what we believe, when someone proposes what is seen as an opposing view, we enter a fight or flight mentality. The fight or flight response is a physiological and psychological reaction to challenging situations. Our defensive mechanisms become alerted, and we struggle with ourselves to decide if we are going to engage in battle and debate over our beliefs (the fight response) or keep quiet and allow the moment to pass (the flight response). Most of the time, I notice people attacking other's beliefs - be it diet, politics, or religion - rather than offering an explanation for their own convictions.

The foods on our plates are as important as the thoughts on our minds. This notion segues to ask the questions: What are your thoughts about food? Do you eat to live or live to eat? Do you eat for taste, or do you eat for health? How well is your thought diet? Do you consciously practice positive thinking and healthy thoughts? When the alarm clock awakes you out of your sleep, do you groan "Ugh" and curse the day or declare "Thank you, God!" for the blessings of a new day? The old proverb, *Change your mind, change your life,* is true. Change is inevitable, though. It will happen with or without our permission. Growth, on the other hand, is optional and requires our consent. It takes a conscious effort to grow. So, when they say, "Change your mind, change your life," I interpret the phrase to mean, "By transforming your mind, you permit growth in your life."

Too often, we entertain the thought of change, but that is about as far as it goes. We end up continuing with what we currently do – even though we know that has not worked for us. You say to yourself, "I need to lose weight." But what is your plan? Instead, you should say, "I am going to practice healthier habits like eating fruit for breakfast." It is easier said than done, but it is worth it. To get different results, you must do something different. "I will start tomorrow." That is not productive. "I will start next week." That is not positive thinking. "I will start in January." That is procrastination. You have to be careful how you talk to yourself.

The unconscious mind will default to your learned thoughts, beliefs, and attitudes. You will keep telling yourself, "not right now" or "I will start later" meanwhile, you will still eat the same foods and think the same thoughts that keep you in the same condition that you say you want to change. Therefore, you must challenge yourself to transform your mind. Train the subconscious mind to have productive thoughts by learning to be consciously present and aware of your mindset. Mindfulness raises the consciousness of your thoughts and actions. Positive affirmations help to stop self-sabotage and negative thinking. That is how you change your psychological diet.

Just as the terms health and fitness are congruent, so are the terms health and wellness. However, these terms are not interchangeable. I have explained that health is being free of disease. Health and fitness are dimensions of wellness. Wellness is the system in which every facet of life operates. Wellness is a state of being. There are eight dimensions of wellness - emotional, intellectual, physical, social, occupational, environmental, financial, and spiritual. Each component is a pillar in our overall well-being. Intellectual wellness is developing the mind to think critically and objectively. Typically, when people go on diets, at some point, they force themselves to do something they hate. Be it going to the gym or eating (or restricting) certain foods. That is counterproductive to their weight loss and health goals. The only way to accomplish those goals is to change their thoughts about health, fitness, and wellness.

Intellectual wellness is an essential aspect of the psychological diet. Imagine being on a diet, and you have gone a few weeks depriving yourself of your favorite foods. You are probably craving them by that time, yet you have still managed to hold out. If I asked you what some of your favorite foods are, you would almost instantly picture some of the foods that you have been resisting. Before provoking you to think of them, you would have been attempting to suppress your thoughts of the foods. This is the way it is with dieting. You try to control your thoughts by suppressing them. The following conversation is a depiction of an internal conflict that a dieting person may have between their inner fit self and their inner fat self:

Fat Self: "I think I want some pizza for lunch today."

Fit Self: "Come on man, you don't need pizza. How about a salad?"

Fat Self: "Salad? That's not going to fill me up. Besides, the pizza restaurant has large 2-toppings for six dollars."

Fit Self: "Eat to live, not live to eat. You're not supposed to eat to get full."

Fat Self: "I've been doing well on my diet. I can have a cheat meal."

Fit Self: "A whole pizza, though? You're only cheating yourself."

Fat Self: "Ok, ok! I will eat the salad. I'm getting extra crotons, though."

Fit Self: "Crotons aren't really good for you, so don't eat too many."

Fat Self: "I am starting to hate this diet."

Was that an accurate interpretation of self-talk? I can relate to that inner struggle as it has played out in my head several times throughout my health and wellness journey. Now, you are mad at yourself because you want pizza but settled for salad. What is likely to happen is that you are going to eat the pizza later – far more than one or two slices - causing you to overeat. By applying intellectual wellness to your diet, you can have your pizza and eat it too. Make your own personal-sized pizza with healthy toppings. Rather than suppressing your thoughts, alter them to fit your health and wellness goals. Controlling your thoughts and changing your habits supports healthy lifestyle changes. That is how you transform your mind, and as a result, you make better choices, which improves your health.

There is a widespread belief that it takes 21 days to form new habits, and 90 days for those habits to become a permanent lifestyle change. I wish it were that easy. But 21 days can be a targeted timeframe to build on the implementation of new habits. Within 21 days of consistency, you could improve your knowledge of health and use that knowledge as a foundation to support your health journey. Once you get to 21 days, strive for 90. After 90 days, keep going. As you work on developing healthier habits, you will rewire your brain to believe and accept these new habits as a way of being. The formation of healthy habits, or any habit, is psychological. They are acquired through repetition, and once acquired, habits become involuntary practices.

Eventually, you will lose track of the days, and your new and improved habits will displace the bad ones. That kind of impulse is known as a "force of habit." In the scholarly analysis, *Making health habitual,* Benjamin Gardner, Phillippa Lally, and Jane Wardle discusses the psychological concepts of forming habits and changing behavior:

> Decades of psychological research consistently show that mere repetition of a simple action in a consistent context leads, through associative learning, to the action being activated upon subsequent exposure to those contextual cues (that is, habitually). Once initiation of the action is 'transferred' to external cues, dependence on conscious attention or motiv-

ational processes is reduced. Therefore, habits are likely to persist even after conscious motivation or interest dissipates. Habits are also cognitively efficient because the automation of common actions frees mental resources for other tasks (2012).

After developing a habit, it becomes second nature - a normal manner of behavior. If the habits formed are healthy ones, it adds to the quality of our lives.

Focusing on calories, macronutrients, and physical exercise is an incomplete outlook of health, wellness, and fitness. Most of the diet programs emphasize target weight goals. They do this by just stopping short of guaranteeing that you will lose a specific amount of weight in a given amount of time. They will say, "lose up to 20 pounds in 2 weeks." You have seen this type of advertisement, but what are their success rates? They may measure success by the number of people who lost five or more pounds. I would want to know how many people kept the weight off after they no longer subscribed to the program. Concentrating on losing weight, counting calories, and food deprivation provoke negative thoughts. If you have pessimistic thoughts about your diet program, it will not work. If you do not enjoy the foods you are eating, it will not work. The way we think and talk to ourselves has a tremendous impact on our lives and livelihood.

Our wellness is comprised of a physical, psychological, and spiritual diet. Positive thoughts produce positive words. Positive words produce positive actions. Our actions can recreate our intrapersonal universe – the inner self. God created the universe with a simple command: "Be." And what he commanded was so. In the same way, we can speak into existence a new attitude that can lead to the best version of ourselves in any aspect of life.

EAT MORE PLANTS

The Lord hath created medicines out of the earth; and he that is wise will not abhor them. **-Ecclesiasticus 38:4**

What is the price of your health? Do you value your money, houses, and cars more than your health? Would you trade good health for a million dollars? What about a billion dollars? If you could have one billion dollars in cash delivered to you in exchange for agreeing to be injected with a strand of a terminal illness, what is your answer? No? Is it because you understand that good health is priceless? It is so valuable that you would go broke trying to restore it if it were to threaten your life. Prescription medications are one of the most common means of treating illnesses. According to the Centers for Medicare & Medicaid, "prescription drug spending increased to $335.0 billion in 2018." Nationally, we are spending hundreds of billions of dollars in health care per year, yet we are not getting healthier. What am I missing?

The foods we regularly eat today will impact our health tomorrow. Rather than eating to live and taking preventive measures to protect our future selves, we rely on medicine to treat us and give us a false sense of physical wellness. Western medications do not cure medical conditions; they treat them. To heal is to restore health. To treat is to manage the illness with the application of medicine and (or) surgery. Just because good health is priceless does not mean it does not come at a price. Health is an investment. The way we eat, think, and interact with our surrounding environment has the most significant impact on our health. There are factors beyond our control that can subject us to poor health. But most times, the inner me is the enemy. Meaning our lifestyle choices, diets, and insufficient knowledge of health causes our bodies to turn against us.

Obesity, heart disease, diabetes, hypertension, and even some cancers are lifestyle diseases. A bad diet - the Standard American Diet - sets up the conditions for disease to take up residents inside of your body. If eating SAD promotes sickness because the acidity causes inflammation, what would eating basic foods do for the body? Basic foods are fruits and vegetables. In their natural form (Non-GMO) they are alkaline. Alkaline foods are anti-inflammatory, and they can reverse the effects of eating SAD foods. How a type of food breaks down inside the body determines if it is acidic or alkaline. Even if it is acidic in its raw state, like limes, it may be alkaline-forming upon digestion. The more basic foods you consume, the better your health can be.

Did you realize that there is a science to the color of fruits and vegetables? They are color-coded according to their functions and benefits. Red fruits and vegetables like tomatoes, watermelon, radishes, and beets protect against heart disease, lowers blood pressure, improves brain function, and reduces the chances of developing cancer.

The blue and purple fruits and vegetables – eggplants, blueberries, blackberries, and purple cabbage – helps improve memory, protect against strokes, heart disease, and reduces inflammation.

The fruits and vegetables in the orange and yellow families such as squash, carrots, bananas, and mangos support bone health, boosts immunity, and promote good skin.

Green leafy vegetables, green beans, avocado, and kiwis are members of the green fruits and vegetables. Green fruit and vegetables support digestive health, helps keep healthy teeth and bones, and builds immune health. The benefits from the different colors of fruits and vegetables are numerous, and they overlap. Each group has essential vitamins and minerals that help sustain good health and wellness.

A plant-based diet has more variability than any other diet. Along with *fasting*, the term *plant-based* has become a health and fitness buzz word. As with health and fitness, there is no one size fits all method of eating a plant-based diet. However, there is a healthy and unhealthy way of following the diet. To get the healthiest benefits out of a plant-based diet, you must make it a part of your way of life. A plant-based diet emphasizes eating foods that are grown from seeds. This includes fruits, vegetables, grains, nuts, seeds, and legumes. Animal products – meats, fats, and dairy - should be limited or avoided. Unhealthy plant-based foods include processed foods like refined and enriched grains, fries and potato chips, and dehydrated or canned fruit with added sugar. Although a plant-based diet is not entirely vegetarian nor vegan, you are regularly choosing to eat most of your foods from plant sources.

I follow a plant-based diet, but I occasionally eat fish. I only eat fish with fins and scales – the clean fish of the sea. Some pescatarians eat shellfish such as lobster and shrimp, and they eat fish without scales like catfish. However, catfish is the pig of the sea, and shrimp is the cockroach of the sea. Except for seafood, pescatarians abstain from eating animal flesh and maintain a plant-based diet.

Flexitarian is a relatively new term used to describe the modern plant-based diet. Flexitarian is also known as a Semi-Vegetarian Diet. For people who are hesitant or unwilling to eliminate meats and other animal products from their diets, following a flexitarian lifestyle may be the way to go. Regardless of your preference for animal products, limiting meat consumption and decreasing your intake of processed foods are key characteristics of a plant-based diet.

If I offered you a diet program that puts you at risk for obesity, chronic illnesses, and inflammation, I suppose that you would not accept that diet because of the health complications that are associated with it. Is that a fair assumption? Yet, millions of people are consuming the Standard American Diet daily without considering its impact on their long-term health. A plant-based diet may be the answer to the Standard American Diet. Replace most of the processed junk with whole foods and include plant-based foods in every meal. Simple, huh? "But where do you get your protein from," questions those who have not gained knowledge of health. I believe the more appropriate question is, "are you getting enough fiber in your diet?" Too often, we rely on anecdotes and hearsay about health rather than researched evidence. Why do you believe that you need so much protein? Who told you that this was true? Point to the scientific evidence.

People are becoming ill because they are overeating protein, fats, and unhealthy carbs. In other words, the health crisis in America is linked to a diet full of meat, animal fats, and refined sugar. Since there is not a massive marketing campaign designed to raise awareness of the need for a high fiber diet, let us see what scientific research says. In their study, *The health benefits of dietary fiber*, Melissa M. Kaczmarczyk, Michael J. Miller, and Gregory G. Freund noted:

> Dietary fiber decreases the risk for type 2 diabetes, cardiovascular disease, and colon cancer by reducing the digestion and absorption of macronutrients and decreasing the contact time of carcinogens within the intestinal lumen. In addition, the United States Food and Drug Administration has approved health claims supporting the role of dietary fiber in the prevention of cancer and coronary heart disease (2012).

James M. Lattimer and Mark D. Haub conducted the study, *Effects of Dietary Fiber and Its Components on Metabolic Health.* It investigates the negative correlation between fiber consumption and some health risks. They highlight two of the health claims that have been approved by the FDA:

> The Food and Drug Administration (FDA) has approved two health claims for dietary fiber. The first claim states that, along with a decreased consumption of fats, an increased consumption of dietary fiber from fruits, vegetables, and whole grains may reduce some types of cancer. The second FDA claim supporting health benefits of [dietary fiber] states that diets low in saturated fat and cholesterol and high in fruits, vegetables and whole-grain, have a decreased risk of leading to coronary heart disease (2010).

The FDA approved these assertions because of the overwhelming evidence that has gained attention in the health and nutrition fields. Fiber has significant health benefits, and the consumption of fiber is essential for a healthy diet.

We focus on the one "benefit" of protein that we know about – **GAINS**. Bigger muscles are the marketing strategy to encourage us to eat more protein. By protein, they mean meat and supple-

ments. But protein is found in plant foods, and it is a better quality of protein than that found in meat. Harvard Health Publishing posted a health watch review titled *Meat or beans: What will you have? Part I: Meat.* The article explains:

> A 5-ounce steak has 300 calories, while a cup of pinto beans has 265. But the steak comes with 44 grams of protein, 120 milligrams of cholesterol, and 12 grams of fat, much of it saturated. In contrast, the beans contain 15 grams of protein, no cholesterol, and only 1 gram of fat, which is polyunsaturated. The steak has no carbohydrates and no fiber; the beans have 26 grams of complex carbohydrates and 15 grams of dietary fiber. The beans have more potassium and less sodium than the steak; the iron content of the two foods is identical, but your body is more efficient at absorbing iron from animal sources. Add the enormous price differential to your comparison, and you'll see that beans are a much better nutritional bargain than steak (2011).

By comparison, beans are a better selection. They are less expensive and promote better health.

You may agree that beans are healthy but argue that eating healthy in general costs too much. Well, let us see about that. Continuing with the beans and steak comparison - A pound of dry beans can feed a family of 6 at around .35 cents per person. Steak, on the other hand, costs at least $4.00 per person for a family of 6. It is much more expensive for the choice cuts. Better health is the value of a plant-based diet. The gains from a plant-based diet are significant to the quality of life. So, what do you have to gain by reducing meat intake and increasing plant intake? In the scientific review, *Adverse Effects Associated with Protein Intake above the Recommended Dietary Allowance for Adults,* Ioannis Delimaris concludes:

> Up to 80% of breast, bowel, and prostate cancers are attributed to dietary practices, and international comparisons show positive associations with a high meat diet. The association, however, seems to have been more consistently found for red meat or processed meat and colorectal cancer. Many adults or even adolescents (especially athletes or bodybuilders) self-prescribe protein supplements and overlook the risks of using them, mainly due to misguided beliefs in their performance-enhancing abilities. Individuals who follow these diets are therefore at risk. Extra protein is not used efficiently by the body and may impose a metabolic burden on the bones, kidneys, and liver. Moreover, high-protein/high-meat diets may also be associated

with increased risk for coronary heart disease due to intakes of saturated fat and cholesterol or even cancer (2013).

The evidence is clear; these are the facts. The overconsumption of processed foods and meats – red meat in particular – have more adverse effects than their proposed health benefits. Tell me again why you need so much protein for your body's functions and muscle growth?

Why eat the same 4 animals – cows, chickens, turkey, and pigs – when there are **at least** 20,000 edible plants? Instead of chicken, rice, and broccoli, try red beans and rice – not the instant crap out of the box. Sauté some squash and zucchini or eggplants to serve with it. Hey, do not knock it until you have tried it. Rather than steak and potatoes, serve up Portobello mushroom caps – seasoned to taste – with baked potatoes and asparagus. It is just a suggestion. Eat green leafy vegetables, try to have 2 or 3 meatless meals per week. Most of us are not eating enough plants. 4 servings of fruits and 5 servings of veggies per day are the **minimum** suggested servings. About 90 percent of Americans are not getting their recommended intake of fruits and vegetables. 90 percent!? That is nearly the entire country. The US population is about 330 million. That means only 10 percent of the population consumes enough fruits and veggies. 10 percent of people equal to 33 million people. The remaining 297 million folks are plant (fiber) deficient. America, we have a problem.

Seven of the top 10 leading causes of death in the United States are chronic diseases that can be prevented or healed with a proper diet. Heart disease, cancer, respiratory diseases, stroke, Alzheimer's disease, diabetes, influenza, and kidney disease are the seven leading chronic illnesses. We all know of someone who have died from some of these diseases. Likewise, we all know people who are experiencing failing health due to having these illnesses. They are taking prescription medications to cover up the symptoms, but are they also changing their diets to heal the body? There's an ancient Ayurvedic proverb that says, " *When diet is wrong, medicine is of no use. When diet is correct, medicine is of no need.*" Read that again.... Ayurvedic is an age-old holistic system which focuses on balancing the mind, body, and spirit – emphasizing the word "holistic." Ancient wisdom suggests that medicine is not useful if your diet is still sick, but with a healthy lifestyle, there is no need for medicine.

Plant foods are made up of vitamins and minerals, and they support every part of our being.

Minerals were put into the earth by God the Creator. Soil is formed by weathered rocks. Weathering causes rocks to break down into small particles that becomes pebbles, soil, and dust. Man was created from *"the dust of the ground"* (Genesis 2:7, NIV). To put this scripture in perspective, understand that the same minerals found in the ground – or earth – are the same ones found in us. Minerals are the connection between humans and earth. Perhaps, this is why Dr. Sebi said, *"The body does not need vitamins. The body need minerals."* The first time I heard this quote, I asked myself, "What's the difference between vitamins and minerals?"

We always hear of the importance of vitamins and even amino acids. When is the last time you can recall there being a push to help people understand the significance of minerals? The difference between the two is vitamins are organic and minerals are inorganic. Vitamins can be destroyed with heat, so cooking foods causes them to lose their vitamin properties. Minerals are in simple form; therefore, they cannot be broken down or lose their value. Think of energy – the first law of thermodynamics states that energy cannot be created or destroyed. It can only be transferred or converted from one form to another. The same is true of minerals.

Iron, potassium, magnesium, and calcium are some of the minerals found in soil. Those same minerals are located in the human body. They support different functions between humans and plants; nonetheless, they are essential for the health and wellness of each. The following paragraph highlights some of roles that a few minerals play in humans and plants. This is not a complete list of minerals nor their functions and benefits.

For humans, iron helps make hemoglobin. Hemoglobin is found in the red blood cells, and it is used to transport oxygen through the body. For plants, iron helps produce chlorophyll and energy within plants. The human benefit of potassium is the proper balancing of fluids and helping to keep a steady heartbeat. Additionally, it supports the transmission of nerve impulses, (the electrical signals across neurons - giving literal meaning to the idea that we are electric) and muscle contractions.

Potassium in plants increases the potency, which helps fight off diseases and improve the quality of the fruit of the plant. Magnesium can regulate blood pressure and convert food into energy. It is necessary for heart health and calcium absorption. Magnesium in the soil is a key element of chlorophyll. Chlorophyll is the green pigment in all green plants, and it is vital for photosynthesis where sunlight is converted to food for the plant.

The benefit of calcium is optimal health for teeth and bones. It also helps the function of muscles and nerves and assists in blood clotting. For plant life, calcium is essential for healthy roots. It supports the growth of roots and root hairs. Root hairs are the stringy extensions of roots, and they absorb water and nutrients from the soil. Calcium also helps in the development of leaves.

God, with his divine, infinite wisdom, put the rocks on the earth to make soil. The soil has nutrients for plants to grow. Rich and fertile soil is required for the land of milk and honey. From the earth, animals graze. From the earth, crops grow. From the earth, man was fashioned. Also, from the earth, man should eat. God said, "I give you every seed-bearing plant on the face of the whole earth and every tree that has fruit with seed in it. They will be yours for food" (Genesis 1:29, NIV). It is no coincidence, then, that eating seeded fruits and veggies provides the minerals needed to support a healthy body. Dr. Sebi explains, "When those minerals have been depleted by the presence of disease, a disease ensues, so you have to replace them in a natural form. In the form of a rock or a plant? A plant because it is alive, and it is electrical. Why does it have to be electrical? Because the body is electrical." Dr. Sebi's diet is highly recommended for holistic health. But even if you are not willing to follow Dr. Sebi's dietary suggestions, I am providing the evidence to show why it is essential to eat more plants. Whether it is in the form of raw whole food, a smoothie, or juice, it does not matter. Just strive to get enough fruits and veggies each day and attempt to transition to a healthy version of a plant-based diet.

PLANNING
FOR HEALTH

"The greatest medicine of all is teaching people how not to need it". — **Hippocrates**

Many years ago, I worked as a waiter at a buffet. Just as the "guest" – hospitality talk for customers – would serve themselves, so did the staff. My co-workers and I would eat throughout the shift. On most nights, some of us would have eaten enough for two by the end of our shift. The restaurant was inside the pavilion area of a riverboat casino. The casino was always hosting different events, and free food was a common ploy to get people to come out.

Many times, we would serve as many people during the week as we would on the weekend. Waiting tables there was a fast-paced job. I am sure 10,000 steps per shift were the minimum number of steps taken by any of the evening shift waiters. Although we frequently indulged in the self-service foods, no one ever seemed to gain any weight. This is not to say that all of us were fit and in shape. Most of us were overweight, but we were not putting on any additional pounds.

Considering the calories in-calories out method, we were burning as many calories as we were consuming, and this held the weight gain in check. In addition to being overweight, some of us had high blood pressure, and others had diabetes. Gastrointestinal problems were a common complaint by my colleagues and me. Several of my coworkers frequently griped about upset stomachs and gas. Constipation and heartburn were also regular ailments that plagued some staff members. I always felt bloated. It was like I was always full, but the stuffed feeling was self-induced. That is the way it is when you are constantly overeating.

The restaurant offered a different dinner theme throughout the week. If my memory is correct, Mondays were all you can eat steak. Tuesday's special was prime rib, and on Wednesdays, baby back ribs were served. My memory may be sketchy on which theme came on which night. However, I am positive that Seafood Extravaganza was on Fridays. It was the busiest night of the week. Perhaps even more than the guests, we dined on fried catfish, shrimp, and unlimited helpings of crab legs and crawfish (when they were in season). Even though we ate so much food, we still expressed concern about our weight. At various times, several of the restaurant employees were trying out different fad diets and weight loss supplements.

As you know by now, I was among those who were trying out different weight loss methods. No one had ever considered that the types of food and how often we were eating them contradicted our weight loss efforts. What was more important is that no one was seriously considering the health complications that were regularly being discussed and complained about. As long as there was medicine to mask the symptoms, no one gave their health a second thought.

After leaving the restaurant business behind, I moved on to a manufacturing company. This was my introduction to 12-hour, rotating shift work. One of the first things I noticed was that nearly all my team members carried huge 24 can coolers for lunch boxes. At the start of the shift, the lunch boxes were full. By the end of the shift, they were on E. As I became acclimated to the culture of the plant, I also carried an extra-large lunch box. I, too, would fill it before work. And by the end of my shift, the cooler that I carried my lunch in would be empty.

There was an extreme change in my daily activity. I went from always being on the move, taking up to 20,000 steps per night as a waiter, to driving forklifts and operating machinery, which earned me roughly a fourth of the number of steps. Meaning, the number of calories I typically burned in the restaurant drastically reduced after I started my career in manufacturing. Because I did not cut my caloric intake, the result was weight gain. This is how I got to be 250 pounds. Excess weight gain was only one problem; declining health was the other. My blood pressure loomed over the hypertension stage. The fatty deposits in my blood vessels that we refer to as cholesterol was dangerously multiplying, and I was at the precipice of being challenged with any number of the health risks that were provoked by my poor dietary habits.

While going through my weight loss journey, I began to understand how to differentiate between fitness, health, and wellness. Each one is different from the other. But they are like coworkers just as the organs of the body are coworkers. They have different functions, but one works in unity with the other for the benefit of the whole body. Illness and disease are insults to the body. The Merriam-Webster dictionary defines the second entry for *insult* as "injury to the body or one of its parts." We injure ourselves with our diets and lifestyle choices.

What we consume or become consumed by either work in favor of or against our fitness, health, and wellness. Being health-conscious and taking proactive measures to be free of biological insults is the proper approach to healthcare. Eating to live, exercising regularly, getting frequent health checkups, and actively engaging in healthy lifestyle habits moves us in the direction of healthcare. In contrast, mindless eating, poor lifestyle choices, a lack of physical activity, and only reacting to illnesses is the sick-care method.

The choices we make about health either support illness or wellness. We are actively planning for one or the other. Both are determined by our lifestyle choices. The cause of the majority of diseases is rooted in lifestyle choices. In the article *Impact of Lifestyle on Health*, Dariush Farhud explains, "According to World Health Organization, 60% of related factors to individual health and quality of life are correlated to lifestyle. Millions of people follow an unhealthy lifestyle. Hence, they encounter illness, disability, and even death. The relationship of lifestyle and health should be highly considered." In the study *Occupational lifestyle diseases: An emerging issue*, Mukesh Sharma and P. K. Majumdar corroborate Farhud's statement. The researchers assert:

> [Various diseases] are preventable, and can be lowered with changes in diet, lifestyle, and environment. Lifestyle diseases characterize those diseases whose occurrence is primarily based on daily habits of people and are a result of an inappropriate relationship of people with their environment. The onset of these lifestyle diseases is insidious, they take years to develop, and once encountered do not lend themselves easily to cure. The main factors contributing to the lifestyle diseases include bad food habits, physical inactivity, wrong body posture, and disturbed biological clock (2009).

Negative lifestyle choices make us more susceptible to the onset of disease than genetics. These problems lead to lifestyle diseases. Each one can be cured with proper health guidance and planning, but more importantly, they are preventable.

Insufficient knowledge of health and inadequate healthcare planning establishes future sick-care. I was on the road to sick-care. The lifestyle habits that I learned early in life had followed me into young adulthood. I was health un-conscious and was expecting the day to come when my family's generational health curses would attach themselves to me. I had to unlearn and relearn to understand why similar health problems seem to systematically attack family members. It is more than family health history. We must consider the diets, lifestyle choices, environment, and habits that family members have in common. Then, we can begin to understand and eliminate the preventable causes of diseases that we mistakenly believe that we are destined to inherit. Furthermore, we will learn that our body weight in general, but specifically the excess body fat we carry, is interrelated to our health.

Obesity is more than a problem with weight, it is a health problem. We focus on weight loss because it is tangible. We can see the results of weight loss. Health, on the other hand, is mostly thought of in the abstract. If we feel fine, then health is a second thought, if it is a thought at all. Sometimes, health complications are not so apparent; they fester and progressively worsen. By the time we start to notice, in some cases, it is already a serious offense to our wellness. We see and feel progressive weight gain, and others notice it too. Just as unhealthy weight gain is a slow process, the same is true for other health-related conditions. We do not just wake up one day and experience health issues. They often become an unintentional part of our lives before we know they are there.

We are busy planning out all other life's events such as education and career goals, and planning our next vacation, but when it comes to health, we can be negligent. It is an oversight on our part. We fail to notice until concerning signs and symptoms began alarming. Then, we respond to the chaos. We seek medical attention and are pre-scribed ointments, pills, and surgery. These things may be necessary to relieve us of imminent dan-ger to our health, but what about changing how we live? The ointments, pills, and surgery are not cures, but they can temporarily sustain us. But to be well, we must make a lifestyle change built upon better health habits.

Planning for health guides us in accomplish-ing the task of improving and maintaining good health. It has to be on our radar, and we have to be diligent in our efforts. To be diligent is to be care-ful. We should treat our health as we would a box that has "fragile" stamped on it. We are ultimately responsible for our own health, however, becom-ing healthy - and maintaining health – requires dedication and discipline. It requires a certain mindset and level of energy that many of us do not have, yet. Just because we do not have it does not mean we should not work to attain it. We must question our lifestyle choices and begin to govern ourselves according to the way we desire to be – assuming that we all wish to be healthy.

Our attitudes toward health as a society reminds me of the tale, The Carpenter's House:

> An elderly carpenter was ready to retire. He told his employer-contractor of his plans to leave the house building business and live a more leisurely life with his wife enjoying his extended family.
>
> He would miss the paycheck, but he needed to retire. They could get by. The contractor was sorry to see his good worker go and asked if he could build just one more house as a personal favor. The carpenter said yes, but in time it was easy to see that his heart was not in his work. He resorted to shoddy workmanship and used inferior materials. It was an unfortunate way to end his career.
>
> When the carpenter finished his work and the builder came to inspect the house, the contractor handed the front-door key to the carpenter. "This is your house," he said, "my gift to you."
>
> What a shock! What a shame! If he had only

known he was building his own house, he would have done it all so differently. Now he had to live in the home he had built none too well.

So, it is with us. We build our lives in a distracted way, reacting rather than acting, willing to put up less than the best. At important points we do not give the job our best effort. Then with a shock we look at the situation we have created and find that we are now living in the house we have built. If we had realized that, we would have done it differently.

Think of yourself as the carpenter. Think about your house. Each day you hammer a nail, place a board, or erect a wall. Build wisely. It is the only life you will ever build. Even if you live it for only one day more, that day deserves to be lived graciously and with dignity. The plaque on the wall says, "Life is a do-it-yourself project." Your life tomorrow will be the result of your attitudes and the choices you make today (n.d.).

Our bodies are the houses that our souls, our energy, the essence of God, lives in. You owe it to yourself and those who love you to strive to maintain a healthy existence. Our lifestyle habits and choices are the materials that we use to sculpt our bodily residence. Eating an unhealthy diet, smoking, drinking excess alcohol, and lacking physical exercise are likened to shoddy workmanship. These bad habits cause inferior health conditions. Then, we are shocked and dismayed when we are handed over the keys to assume ownership of our unhealthy dwelling, albeit we were the builders of it.

Prevention is the most effective and practical way to improve health. By taking preventive measures, we must actively plan and prep instead of being passive about our diet and health. It keeps our health at the forefront of our minds. Planning for health helps us to minimize our intake of processed foods and replace them with natural healthy foods. Pauline Ducrot, Caroline Méjean, and others published their research on the potential benefits of meal planning in the *International Journal of Behavioral Nutrition and Physical Activity*. Their findings "highlighted that individuals planning their meals were more likely to have a better dietary quality, including a higher adherence with nutritional guidelines as well as an increased food variety. Additionally, meal planning was associated with lower odds of being obese in men and women." Meal planning and prepping help to correct the imbalance between calories-in and calories-out and causes us to think in advance of what we will eat for the next several days.

Practicing this habit sets into motion a mind-set shift that becomes open to relearning all that you thought you knew about health, wellness, and weight loss.

Planning for health drives us to renew our attitudes towards eating healthy foods, engaging in physical activity, and managing stress. We are encouraged to figure out ways to become more active and abandon the old sedentary lifestyle that we have persisted in living. Similarly, we will hold ourselves accountable by rejecting the negative affirmations that we routinely tell ourselves. The planning and prepping process helps to find reasons to commit to your overall general health.

To transform your health, you have to transform your mind. Most people know the importance of healthy living, yet they lack the wisdom and understanding of embodying such a mindset. They settle for a "we have to die from something" kind of thinking. Yet, when the repercussions of poor lifestyle choices start to manifest as sickness and disease, they expect doctors to treat and prolong the life that they have been neglectful with. It is simple enough to set health and wellness goals and work toward positive incremental changes. Setting specific, measurable, attainable, realistic, and timely (SMART) goals can keep you inspired and motivated to start and continue your health, wellness, and weight loss goals. The article *Wellness Coaching to Improve Lifestyle Behaviors Among Adults With Prediabetes* discuss how goal setting supports a healthy lifestyle. The authors, Ramona S. DeJesus, MD, Matthew M. Clark, Ph.D., Lila J. Finney Rutten, Ph.D., and others advise, "Goal setting skills are crucial to engage in positive behavior change; problem-solving skills in contrast are essential to maintaining positive behavioral changes. Enhanced goal setting skills translates to increased self-efficacy which then promotes healthy lifestyle behavior in both diet and physical activity." Meal planning and prepping and setting SMART goals are methods to combat the sick-care system. Planning for health is an intentional way to administer self-control and aim for a lifestyle that promotes wellness.

FINAL WEIGH-IN

Knowledge of health is the foundation of a healthy lifestyle. Before you can apply knowledge, you must attain it first. Without knowledge, there is no wisdom because you cannot apply what you do not know. Knowledge of health means becoming aware of how your physical, mental, and spiritual diets affect your overall health. When we know better, we are then obligated to do better. Applying knowledge is wisdom, and wisdom brings forth understanding.

The miseducation of dieting has caused an epidemic of chronic illnesses. Obesity is steadily increasing along with portion sizes. Eating fast food several times a week is a way of life now. When we order the fast food, we say, "Well, the large only cost an extra .40 cents more." This is the first generation where parents are predicted to outlive their children due to the rise of obesity and health care issues that are starting during childhood. People prescribe themselves to weight loss diets as a solution to their problem. Yet, the problem persists. We are more concerned about our weight than our health. A slender frame is not indicative of better health. Nor does a muscular build indicates that an individual is healthy. Slim and (or) muscular persons can be just as unhealthy as an obese person if their diet is not well. I do not intend to downplay the importance of weight loss and maintaining a healthy weight – "healthy" being the keyword. However, successful weight loss is often sabotaged because of the emphasis that we put on the numbers on the scale.

Focusing on weight loss is counterproductive to health gains. Living a healthy lifestyle and eating well is the way to lose weight. Instead, people will sacrifice their health and wellness to shed pounds. The health goal, as it relates to weight loss, is to lose fat. You can lose a substantial amount of weight due to illnesses. The effects of diabetes or some cancers can cause a considerable reduction in body weight. Weight loss can be a combination of losing muscle, water, and fat, whereas fat loss is just that – losing excesses fat.

Expecting to lose ten pounds a week is an unrealistic expectation. Losing that much weight that fast is almost guaranteed to be an unhealthy combination of water, muscle, and fat loss. Guess what, though? The irony of this kind of weight loss effort is ultimately weight gain. Once you stop the extreme dieting, the weight returns. And in most cases, the weight comes back with about 10 – 15 friends. When people lose weight like this, it is a vain weight loss. It is done for conceited reasons, thereby being unsuccessful. To accomplish this kind of slimming, people turn to weight loss challenges, smoothie cleanses, diet pills, counting calories, intermittent fasting (as a diet), and restricting carbs. But it does not work. When the phase is over, then what? It is causing an unhealthy cycle of yo-yo dieting with fruitless results. There must be a lifestyle change to get long-term effects.

Have you ever heard anyone say they are trying to "build lean muscle?" Maybe, you have said it yourself. I am guilty of it too. Putting on "lean muscle" is a misnomer because all muscle is lean. When someone says this, what they are referring to is trimming the fat. To be lean is to have very little fat. Therefore, lean has more to do with fat loss than it does muscle gain. Think about when you buy meat from the grocery store. The leaner meats have less fat. When we do not have excess fat, our bodies are more efficient and burn more calories throughout the day. Without the extra fat, we can expect a better quality of life. So, to carry excess fat predisposes us to disease. To say disease is hereditary is a cop-out that allows us to accept the conditions that are making our family members meet an untimely death. You can get the best out of your DNA simply by following a healthy lifestyle.

We are all on a health journey. It is either in the direction of good or bad health. Not practicing clean eating, following the Standard American Diet, not fasting or cleansing regularly all contributes to a journey of bad health. The consequences are sickness, obesity, and precious years taken from your life. Even if the effects of a bad diet are not outwardly evident to you, the long-term health effects are clandestinely shaping inside of you. It is similar to how termites build and destroy. They build their mounds in secret, and you are unaware of the damage until it has been done. If you do not get rid of them soon enough, they will cause more damage. You know if you need to make a change; no one has to convince you of that. It is hard to get started, and it's harder to stay committed. If you are struggling with your weight and health, it's time to begin your journey to good health. How do you start the journey and remain consistent? In closing, I offer you the three pillars that have guided me along with my health, wellness, and weight loss journeys.

Pillar One: *Commit to the Journey*

Make up your mind that you want better health.

You cannot move forward until you have decided that you really want to improve your quality of life and strive for better health. You have to find the reason why you will commit to change. Your why is your purpose – journeys cannot be successful without a purpose. Without meaning, you will not find any value in the journey. I wanted better health because I did not want to go through what I witnessed my mom go through. My "why" was simple. I wanted to live. My mom's near-death experience gave me a renewed perspective on the value of a healthy lifestyle. I do not just want to exist; I want to live and enjoy life.

As with any journey, you need to know where you are coming from to understand where you are going. Concerning health, an excellent way to get an understanding of where you're coming from is to get a health checkup. You need to know your blood pressure numbers, how much fat is in your blood, and the efficiency of your overall bodily functions. What is your weight? Is it a healthy weight? Do not confuse a healthy weight with the BMI ranges. The BMI chart is not exact, but it serves as a good guideline. The best way to know if you are within a healthy weight range is to know your body fat percent. Consult with your doctor annually for a health and wellness diagnostics.

Pillar Two: *Practice Healthy Habits*

Practicing healthy habits such as intermittent fasting and morning or evening jogs supports a healthy lifestyle. If you cannot jog, then walk. We get in the habit of doing things because of the reward that we associate with the habit. One of my favorite books is *The Power of Habit* by Charles Duhigg. In his book, Duhigg provides several examples of the habit-loop. The habit-loop is comprised of a cycle of cues, routines, and rewards that causes us to do the things that we habitual do. Health is not only a condition of living, but it's also something that we do. Our lifestyle choices, diets and habits lean us toward or away from good health. The goal should be to make more of the choices that lean us toward good health.

To be conscious of your habits, keep a journal of your day to day activities. You can use a notebook, tablet, or cell phone. This can be an arduous task at first, but you should take out some time throughout the day to capture your thoughts and feelings. Notice how you feel and what you are thinking each time you decided to eat. Were you hungry? Really? Or were you board, and having a snack broke the monotony of a mundane task? When you have lunch, is it because you have identified a particular time of day as a cue to eat, or are you actually hungry? As you continue to write down these things, you will begin to see a pattern emerge. Then, you will become aware of some of your problem habits. Once you are aware of what is causing you to do the unhealthy things you do, you can work on improving the bad habit.

Being consistent in practicing healthy habits leads to lifestyle changes. Healthy lifestyle changes lead to a new and better version of you. To improve your old habits requires practice. Habits are like muscles. You must work them out to make them grow. The more you focus on and practice healthier habits, the more they become a part of your way of life.

Pillar Three: Stop Going on Diets

Diets do not work. Diets are seen as quick-fix solutions to the obesity crisis. Although they have proven to fail time after time, diets are still the preferred method to lose weight. Diet, as the way it was intended to mean, adds value to the complex systems of health and wellness. However, diet, as the way it is interrupted, causes an unhealthy concept of weight and body image which imposes a negative dieting mindset on people who struggle with their weight.

Stop dieting and starting healthing. The focus should always be on how you feel, not how much you weigh. If you can commit to make healthcare and health awareness an active part of your daily life, you will inevitably make food and lifestyle choices that support a healthy you. By doing so, the excess weight will be lost and not found again.

Your journey will not be identical to mine. You will not need to do exactly as I did. There are different routes to get there. The objective is to get there. 4+3 = 7 and so does 5+2. These pillars are suggestive methods – recommended courses of action - to help improve health and wellness, which can lead to a healthy lifestyle that supports healthy weight loss.

REFERENCES

Alberts, B. (1970, January 1). How Cells Obtain Energy from Food. Retrieved from https://www.ncbi.nlm.nih.gov/books/NBK26882/

American College of Cardilology. (2018, July 23). Cover Story: Obesity and Cardiovascular Disease Risk. Retrieved from https://www.acc.org/latest-in-cardiology/articles/2018/07/06/12/42/cover-story-obesity-and-cardiovascular-disease-risk

American Heart Association. (2013). High Blood Pressure. Retrieved July 2019, from https://www.heart.org/idc/groups/heart-public/@wcm/@sop/@smd/documents/downloadable/ucm_319587.pdf

American Heart Association. (n.d.). Knowing No Bounds: Stroke in Infants, Children, and Youth. Retrieved September 2020, from https://www.heart.org/-/media/files/about-us/policy-research/fact-sheets/facts-stoke-in-infants-children-youth.pdf?la=en&hash=FDCA15F64A10AEDA77D5C2C7AC5CFCCD74AE28EE

American Psychological Association. (2013). How stress affects your health. Retrieved from https://www.apa.org/helpcenter/under-standing-chronic-stress

American Public Media. (n.d.). American RadioWorks - Say it Plain, Say it loud. Retrieved July 2019, from http://americanradioworks.publicradio.org/features/black-speech/mx.html

Anton, S. D., Moehl, K., Donahoo, W. T., Marosi, K., Lee, S. A., Mainous, A. G., ... Mattson, M. P. (2018, February). Flipping the Metabolic Switch: Understanding and Applying the Health Benefits of Fasting. Retrieved from https://www.ncbi.nlm.nih.gov/pubmed/29086496

Begley, S. (2008, November 12). Train Your Mind, Change Your Brain. Retrieved from https://books.google.com/books?id=U5XNEQadiU8C&lpg=PA7&ots=n85k-FBb-b1&dq=change your mind change your life&lr&pg=PA9#v=onepage&q=brain&f=false

Big Breakfast®: Full Breakfast Meal: McDonald's. (n.d.). Retrieved November 2019, from https://www.mcdonalds.com/us/en-us/product/big-breakfast.html

Bloomer, R. J., Kabir, M. M., Canale, R. E., Trepanowski, J. F., Marshall, K. E., Farney, T. M., & Hammond, K. G. (2010, September 3). Effect of a 21 day Daniel Fast on metabolic and cardiovascular disease risk factors in men and women. Retrieved from https://www.ncbi.nlm.nih.gov/pubmed/20815907/

Bollow, J. (2009). How Fast is Your Brain? Retrieved August 3, 2019, from https://

thephenomenalexperience.com/content/how-fast-is-your-brain

Cedars Sinai. (n.d.). Hemorrhagic Stroke. Retrieved March 6, 2020, from https://www.cedars-sinai.edu/Patients/Health-Conditions/Hemorrhagic-Stroke.aspx

Center for Chronic Disease Prevention. (2020, January 31). Stroke Facts. Retrieved February 2020, from https://www.cdc.gov/stroke/facts.htm

Center for Chronic Disease Prevention. (2019, December 2). Heart Disease Facts. Retrieved from https://www.cdc.gov/dhdsp/data_statistics/fact_sheets/fs_heart_disease.htm

Centers for Medicare & Medicaid Services. (2020, March 24). NHE Fact Sheet. Retrieved from https://www.cms.gov/Research-Statistics-Data-and-Systems/Statistics-Trends-and-Reports/NationalHealthExpend-Data/NHE-Fact-Sheet

Collingwood, J. (2018, October 8). The Psychology of Diets. Retrieved February 29, 2020, from https://psychcentral.com/lib/the-psychology-of-diets/

DeJesus, R. S., Clark, M. M., Rutten, L., Hathaway, J. C., Wilson, P. M., Link, S. M., & Sauver, J. S. (2018). Wellness Coaching to Improve Lifestyle Behaviors Among Adults With Prediabetes: Patients' Experience and Perceptions to Participation. *Journal of patient experience*, 5(4), 314–319. https://doi.org/10.1177/2374373518769118

Delimaris, I. (2013, July 18). Adverse Effects Associated with Protein Intake above the ... Retrieved from https://www.hindawi.com/journals/isrn/2013/126929/

Dictionary.com, LLC. (n.d.). Lifestyle disease. Retrieved from https://www.dictionary.com/browse/lifestyle-disease

Ducrot, P., Méjean, C., Aroumougame, V., Ibanez, G., Allès, B., Kesse-Guyot, E., Hercberg, S., & Péneau, S. (2017). Meal planning is associated with food variety, diet quality and body weight status in a large sample of French adults. *The international journal of behavioral nutrition and physical activity*, *14*(1), 12. https://doi.org/10.1186/s12966-017-0461-7

Farhud D. D. (2015). Impact of Lifestyle on Health. *Iranian journal of public health*, *44*(11), 1442–1444.

Fry, T. (n.d.). Quotes by T.C. Fry. Retrieved April 13, 2020, from https://www.goodreads.com/author/show/706795.T_C_Fry

Gardner, B., Lally, P., & Wardle, J. (2012). Making health habitual: the psychology of 'habit-formation' and general practice. *The British journal of general practice: the journal of the Royal College of General Practitioners*, *62*(605), 664–666. https://doi.org/10.3399/bjgp12X659466

GI Disorders Functional GI Disorders Motility Disorders Upper GI Disorders Lower GI Disorders Other Disorders Kids &

Teens. (2019, October). Retrieved August 2020, from https://www.iffgd.org/manage-your-health/the-digestive-system.html

Harvard Health Publishing. (2011, February). Meat or beans: What will you have? Part I: Meat. Retrieved March 1, 2020, from https://www.health.harvard.edu/staying-healthy/meat-or-beans-what-will-you-have-part-i-meat

Harvard Health Publishing. (2015, February). The truth about fats: the good, the bad, and the in-between. Retrieved January 2020, from https://www.health.harvard.edu/staying-healthy/the-truth-about-fats-bad-and-good

HHS Office, & Council on Sports. (2017, January 26). Facts & Statistics. Retrieved from https://www.hhs.gov/fitness/resource-center/facts-and-statistics/index.html

Holland, K. (2020, March 9). Obesity Facts in America. Retrieved May 23, 2020, from https://www.healthline.com/health/obesity-facts#1

Kaczmarczyk, M. M., Miller, M. J., & Freund, G. G. (2012, August). The health benefits of dietary fiber: beyond the usual suspects of type 2 diabetes mellitus, cardiovascular disease and colon cancer. Retrieved from https://www.ncbi.nlm.nih.gov/pmc/articles/PMC3399949/

Kallem, S., Carroll-Scott, A., Gilstad-Hayden, K., Peters, S. M., McCaslin, C., & Ickovics, J. R. (2013, June). Children's report of lifestyle counseling differs by BMI status. Retrieved from https://

www.ncbi.nlm.nih.gov/pmc/articles/
PMC3727518/

Krispy Kreme Doughnuts. (2016, March 2). Original Glazed Doughnuts. Retrieved October 22, 2019, from http://kkd-nutritional-panels.s3.amazonaws.com/2018Original-GlazedDoughnutRetailPanel.pdf

Lattimer, M., J., Haub, & D., M. (2010, December 15). Effects of Dietary Fiber and Its Components on Metabolic Health. Retrieved from https://www.mdpi.com/2072-6643/2/12/1266/htm

Lerma-Cabrera, J.M., Carvajal, F. & Lopez-Legarrea, P. Food addiction as a new piece of the obesity framework. *Nutr J* **15**, 5 (2015). https://doi.org/10.1186/s12937-016-0124-6

Lexico. (n.d.). Diet: Definition of Diet by Lexico. Retrieved from https://www.lexico.com/en/definition/diet

Lexico. (n.d.). Obesity: Definition of Obesity by Lexico. Retrieved from https://www.lexico.com/en/definition/obesity

Lindberg, S., & Murrell, D. (2018, August 23). Autophagy: What You Need to Know. Retrieved March 24, 2020, from https://www.healthline.com/health/autophagy

Mark, J. J. (2020, April 7). Imhotep. Retrieved from https://www.ancient.eu/imhotep/

Merriam-Webster. (n.d.). Disease. Retrieved from https://www.merriam-webster.com/dictionary/disease

Merriam-Webster. (n.d.). Insult. Retrieved from https://www.merriam-webster.com/dictionary/insult

National Cancer Institute. (n.d.). Cancer of Any Site - Cancer Stat Facts. Retrieved December 2019, from https://seer.cancer.gov/statfacts/html/all.html

National Cancer Institute. (2018, April 27). Cancer Statistics. Retrieved from https://www.cancer.gov/about-cancer/understanding/statistics

Online Etymology Dictionary. (n.d.). health (n.). Retrieved from https://www.etymonline.com/word/health

Online Etymology Dictionary. (n.d.). -th. Retrieved from https://www.etymonline.com/word/-th

Online Etymology Dictionary. (n.d.). dis-. Retrieved from https://www.etymonline.com/word/dis-

Online Etymology Dictionary. (n.d.). ease (n.). Retrieved from https://www.etymonline.com/word/ease

Saturated Fat. (n.d.). Retrieved from https://www.heart.org/en/healthy-living/healthy-eating/eat-smart/fats/saturated-fats

Sharma, M., & Majumdar, P. K. (2009). Occupational lifestyle diseases: An emerging issue. *Indian journal of occupational and environmental medicine, 13*(3), 109–112. doi:10.4103/0019-5278.58912

Sodium: How to tame your salt habit. (2019, June 29). Retrieved from https://www.mayo-clinic.org/healthy-lifestyle/nutrition-and-healthy-eating/in-depth/sodium/art-20045479

The African Bio-mineral Balance. (2018, September 21). Dr. Sebi on Vita-mins and Mineral (Must Watch) "The African Bio-Mineral Balance. Retrieved from http://theafricanbiomineralbalance.com/dr-sebi-on-vitamins-and-mineral-must-watch/

The American Institute of Stress. (2020, March 24). What is Stress? Retrieved from https://www.stress.org/

The Carpenter's House. (n.d.). Retrieved from http://www.inspirationpeak.com/cgi-bin/stories.cgi?record=22

The Editors of Encyclopedia Britannica. (2019, November 11). Imhotep. Retrieved from https://www.britannica.com/biography/Imhotep

Welcome, A. (2019, August 29). Definition of Obesity. Retrieved from https://obesitymedicine.org/definition-of-obesity/

What is High Blood Pressure? (n.d.). Retrieved from https://www.heart.org/en/health-topics/high-blood-pressure/the-facts-about-high-blood-pressure/what-is-high-blood-pressure

www.myfitnesspal.com. (n.d.). Retrieved from https://www.myfitnesspal.com/food/calories/

gala-apple-120-g-red-apple-me-
dium-384875721

ABOUT THE AUTHOR

T. M. 'Lijah

Psychology major, aspiring health coach, author, and teacher, T. M. 'Lijah is a health and wellness advocate. After being challenged with obesity, high blood pressure, and other ailments, T. M. 'Lijah became self-taught on the aspects of physical, mental, and spiritual health. As he gained knowledge of health, he lost nearly 100 pounds and improved his overall wellness. T. M. 'Lijah lives in the Shreveport - Bossier area of Louisiana.

Made in the USA
Middletown, DE
02 November 2022

13944422R00099